1. **This book may be kept three weeks. It is to be returned on / before the last date stamped below.**
2. **A fine of 25c will be charged for every week or part of week a book is overdue.**

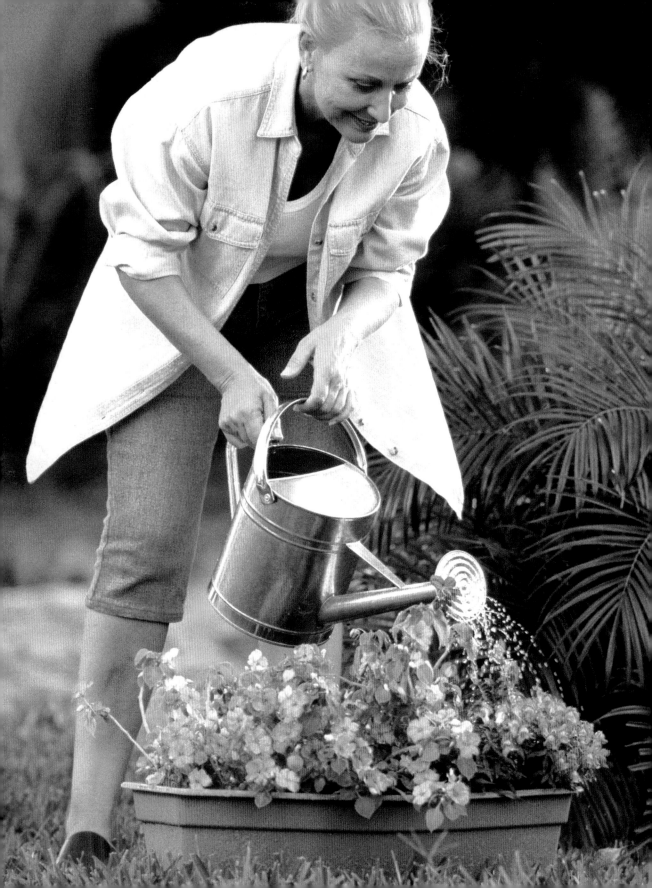

Overcoming
arthritis

A holistic plan including a unique tai chi programme
to relieve pain and restore mobility

Dr. Paul Lam & Judith Horstman

A Dorling Kindersley Book

London, New York, Munich, Melbourne, Delhi

Project Editor: Pip Morgan
Project Designer: Phil Gamble
Senior Editor: Penny Warren
Senior Art Editor: Margherita Gianni
Managing Editor: Stephanie Farrow
Managing Art Editor: Mabel Chan
Production Controller: Sarah Dodd
DTP Designer: Karen Constanti
Jacket Design: Chris Drew, Mark Cavanagh

First published in Great Britain in 2002 by
Dorling Kindersley Limited,
80 Strand, London WC2R 0RL

A Penguin Company
2 4 6 8 10 9 7 5 3 1

Reproduced in Italy by GRB Editrice s.r.l
Printed and bound in Spain

See our complete catalogue at www.dk.com

IMPORTANT NOTICE
Do not try self-diagnosis or attempt self-treatment
for serious or long-term problems without
consulting a medical professional or qualified
practitioner. Do not undertake any self-treatment
while you are undergoing a prescribed course of
medical treatment without first seeking professional
advice. Always seek medical advice if symptoms
persist. Do not exceed any dosages recommended
without professional guidance.

CHINESE SPELLING
The Chinese government has been unifying Chinese
spelling in English over recent years. The official
method is called *pin yin*, which means the spelling is
based on the way the words sound. Tai chi is the
old spelling which should now be *taijiquan* or *taiji*.
This book uses the *pin yin* method of spelling
Chinese words except for tai chi and *I Ching*, which
are so ingrained. Chi is spelled *qi*, chi kung is
qigong and dantien is *dan tian*.

Contents

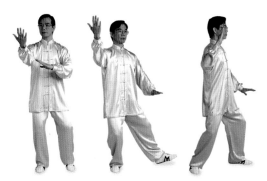

FOREWORD

Most people have heard of arthritis. Many assume it is an inevitable part of getting old and that they will just have to live with the pain and loss of mobility it may bring. But there are many types of arthritis, it can affect people of any age and, while there is no cure for the condition, there are many things people can do to manage arthritis and reduce the negative effects of the pain, fatigue and limitation of movement they may experience.

Alongside conventional medication, people with arthritis use techniques including diet, complementary therapies and exercise to help control their arthritis and keep as healthy and active as possible.

Exercise may seem an unlikely option for people who experience a lot of pain and stiffness. People may be put off by fear of hurting their joints. But sensible exercise boosts energy, helps maintain mobility, keeps muscles supporting the joints strong and encourages relaxation. Tai chi is a safe and gentle form of exercise for people with arthritis. It can be done by people of any age and any fitness level. Importantly, it also has positive effects on relaxation and mental well-being, which are all important in managing pain and achieving a happy and healthy lifestyle.

Dr. Lam's Tai Chi programme has been specially designed for people with arthritis and positive results have been reported by participants throughout the world. Arthritis Care is delighted to support this book and introduce a programme of exercise that we think will be very beneficial to a lot of people with arthritis.

Gill Dorer
Arthritis Care

Introduction

Arthritis in its many forms is one of the most common chronic conditions faced by people worldwide. No one knows for sure how many people have the different kinds of arthritis or related musculoskeletal conditions, but estimates suggest it affects about one in six – nearly a billion people.

In developed countries, arthritis is the number one cause of disability for people over the age of 65, and a major financial burden on healthcare. But the human cost of coping with the pain, stiffness and disability of arthritis can be even greater. And since there is no cure for most kinds of arthritis, many people become depressed, thinking there is nothing they can do about their condition and so resign themselves to a life of restricted activity. That's too bad. Because there are various treatments that can help. And studies show that people who take an active role in the treatment of their illness can improve their quality of life.

This book presents an overview to help you better understand arthritis and what you can do about it. It includes a review of different kinds of arthritis, conventional treatments, options for self–help, lifestyle guidance and complementary treatments that show medical promise.

It features the Tai Chi for Arthritis programme, a series of safe and gentle exercises developed specifically for people with arthritis by a family physician, tai chi instructors, a physiotherapist and two rheumatologists (*see page 144*). The programme does not require deep knee bends and contains qigong, which is a practice especially beneficial for healing and relaxation. People of almost any physical condition or age can learn the programme easily and quickly, and use it to ease the pain and stiffness of arthritis.

More than 60,000 people have learned the programme from trained instructors in association with arthritis foundations – and there is an 80-minute video available (*see page 139*). The result is remarkable. In surveys, 90 per cent of participants say the programme relieved their symptoms and brought about the following effects: relief from pain and stiffness and a lifting of mood; relaxation and tranquillity; and increased flexibility and muscle strength.

Encouraged by these results, medical experts are conducting scientific studies into the beneficial effects of tai chi on arthritis.

Paul Lam MBBS, FAMAC

Paul Lam is a family doctor in Sydney, Australia, who took up tai chi more than 25 years ago to reduce the impact of arthritis on his life. He has gained good control of his arthritis and has become very proficient in tai chi over the years, winning a Gold Medal at the Third International Tai Chi Competition held in Beijing in 1993.

Dr. Lam has taught many people tai chi at the Better Health Tai Chi Chuan Academy in Sydney and in workshops worldwide. He is internationally known for his books and videos about tai chi. His Tai Chi for Arthritis "Train the Trainer" courses for tai chi instructors, exercise leaders, physiotherapists, and qualified movement teachers continue to be in demand at many arthritis foundations.

How Paul Lam discovered tai chi

"When I was a young medical student, I suffered from frequent aches in my neck and back but never thought much about them. Around the time I was about to graduate I noticed the pains were becoming more frequent, and I suddenly realised I had

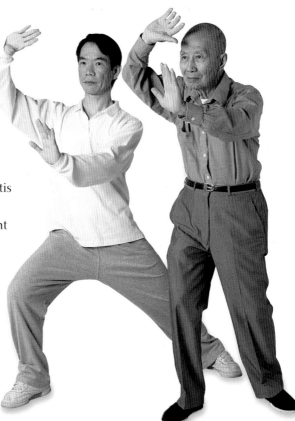

DR. PAUL LAM AND MR. WIN GWAI LUM

the first signs of osteoarthritis. I consulted an orthopaedic specialist who confirmed my self-diagnosis, and disposed of me with a prescription for a powerful non-steroidal anti-inflammatory drug (NSAID). He gave the impression there was nothing to be done and did not offer any advice for dealing with either the pain or the increasing cartilage loss.

"Like most people I went through the emotions of denial, anger and acceptance. Although I was young, arthritis was already affecting my life. I had just tried skiing and loved it. But after a ski weekend, I was in agony. I wanted something to control my arthritis and so enable me to continue skiing and remain active.

"At that time, few realized that exercise can help people with arthritis. In fact, many believed osteoarthritis was made worse by it. But I remembered tai chi was used in China for centuries for many ailments, including arthritis, so I had to try it.

"My first serious teacher turned out to be my father-in-law, Mr. Win Gwai (Frederick) Lum, who is 89 and still enjoying excellent health. He encouraged me to find the best teachers, and I studied for many years with Professor Men Hui Feng and his wife Professor Kan Gui Xiang from the Beijing University of Physical Education.

"I discovered that tai chi does wonderful things. The immediate effect is that no matter how anxious or tired I was, after practising I felt good all over. My mind became clear and my body felt great. The long-term effect became obvious later.

Gradually, I saw improvements in my mental concentration, ability to relax and overall fitness level. I became an enthusiastic student. Now in my 50s, my arthritis is well under control. I easily out-endure most of my ski partners. I used to avoid living in a house with stairs because going up and down would always hurt. For the last 14 years we've lived in a house with three flights.

"I founded the Better Health Tai Chi Chuan Academy in Sydney where I have my medical practice. Some years ago, I began to make teaching and demonstration videos about tai chi. I realized that I wanted to share this wonderful art with other people with arthritis."

Judith Horstman

Judith Horstman is an award-winning journalist who writes about health and medicine for doctors as well as the general public. She is the author of the Arthritis Foundation's Guide to Alternative Therapies, and a contributing editor for *Arthritis Today*, the magazine of the Arthritis Foundation of the United States.

Her work has appeared in hundreds of publications worldwide, including many Internet sites. She has been a Washington correspondent and a journalism professor and received a Knight Science Journalism Fellowship at MIT (Massachusetts Institute of Technology). She has also received two Fulbright awards to teach journalism in Budapest, Hungary.

Ms. Horstman has practised meditation and yoga for more than 25 years, and is a tai chi student of Dr. Paul Lam. She lives in San Francisco, California, near her children and grandchildren.

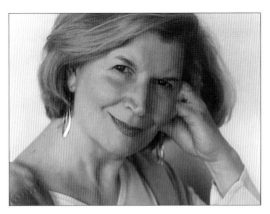

JUDITH HORSTMAN

How Judith Horstman found tai chi

"All of my life I have been blessed with good health and have been very active. I enjoyed horseback riding, camping, hiking, dance, yoga, skiing, house renovations, gardening and travel. But a motor vehicle accident a few years ago changed all that.

"Suddenly, I was in such pain that I couldn't sleep or function properly without drugs. I could not play with my toddler granddaughter or even carry my new-born grandsons. Along with other injuries, doctors discovered that my sacroiliac joint (in the lower back) was injured and that I had osteoarthritis in my back and neck.

"Nonetheless, I expected I would soon return to my previous active life without the drugs and therapy. I had physical therapy, acupuncture, massage and treatment at a chronic pain clinic. Since I had practised yoga and meditation for 30 years, I returned to these practices with renewed commitment.

"But the chronic pain from the sacroiliac joint did not improve, and most exercises – even yoga – brought me more pain. When

a rehabilitation expert told me that I would probably always need to take some drugs or treatment, and that my osteoarthritis would most likely get worse as a result of the injuries I sustained in the accident, I became very depressed.

"In the midst of this, I was writing my book about alternative therapies for arthritis. I discovered Paul Lam's Tai Chi for Arthritis programme and found I could do it without pain. The tai chi helps to relieve the stiffness without stressing my injured sacroiliac joint or the osteorthritis in my neck and back, and the meditative power of the tai chi programme renews my inner core of calmness.

"I then had the great good fortune to meet Paul Lam, and to begin working with him both as a student of tai chi and as joint authors of this book.

"Today, I try to practise what I write about. I control my musculoskeletal pain with a combination of mild exercises and Western medical treatments along with less conventional therapies, such as meditation and tai chi.

"I know that maintaining this routine may help to keep my osteoarthritis from getting worse. But best of all, it helps keep me strong so that I can look forward to many active years with my grandchildren."

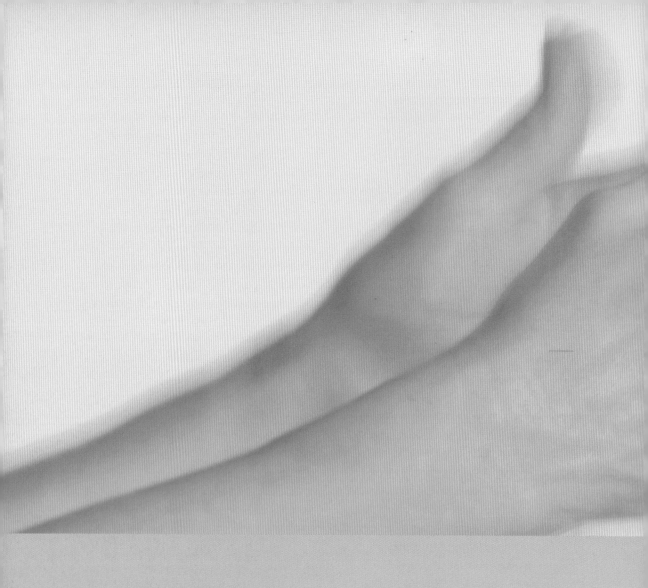

Arthritis
explained

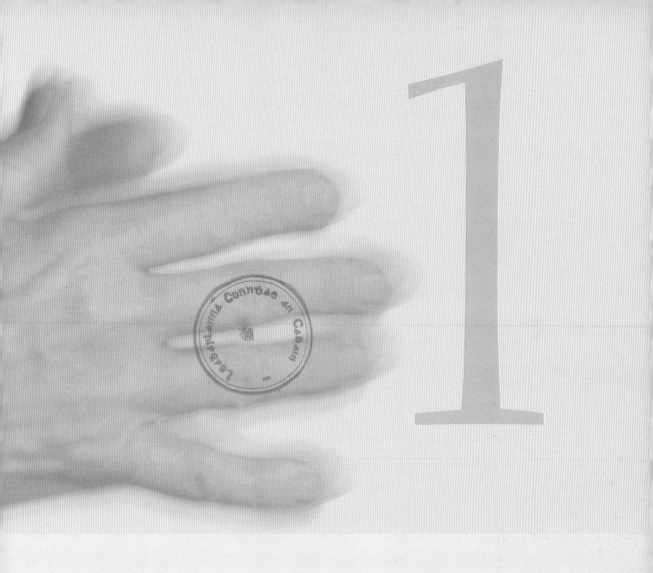

The symptoms and severity of arthritis range from a mild form, controlled without medicine or with over-the-counter pain relievers, to a disabling and even life-threatening disease that causes severe pain and can drastically change your life.

What is arthritis?

Arthritis in its many forms is one of the most common chronic conditions in developed countries. It is also a worldwide health problem, affecting as many as one billion people of every age, race and culture. Arthritis is not a new disease. Skeletal remains show humans had arthritis in 4,500 BC and even some dinosaur bones show evidence of arthritic damage.

There are more than 100 kinds of arthritis and related conditions. The word arthritis comes from *arthr* (joint) and *itis* (inflammation). It is used to describe a wide range of diseases of the joints and related tissues that cause pain, stiffness and sometimes joint deformities and loss of function. Some kinds of arthritis also attack the skin and internal organs. You may have heard arthritis referred to as rheumatism or rheumatic disease: the terms are used interchangeably and arthritis specialists are called rheumatologists.

The risk of getting many kinds of arthritis increases as we age. Today, joint diseases account for half of all chronic conditions in people aged 60 and older. Because medicine and diet are helping us live longer, more people than ever will develop osteoarthritis in the future. But other forms of arthritis also attack children and people in the prime of life. Some of these rheumatic diseases, such as rheumatoid arthritis, lupus and ankylosing spondylitis, are very serious.

Diagnosing and treating arthritis

Arthritis can be a complex condition to diagnose and treat. Many people, especially as they age, develop osteoarthritis in addition to other kinds of arthritis, or are also being treated for other chronic diseases, such as heart disease or diabetes. Moreover, because no two individuals have exactly the same symptoms, your doctor will most likely prescribe a combination of treatments adjusted specifically for you. A team approach is recommended for treating the more severe types of arthritis. When treating chronic ailments, doctors today are increasingly open to the idea of including some complementary therapies (*see Chapters Two and Three*).

The cause of most kinds of arthritis is not known, nor is there a cure for the majority of them. But many symptoms do respond to treatment. By working closely with your healthcare team and using a combination of conventional medications, complementary therapies and exercise, you can minimize the effects of this age–old disease and remain active.

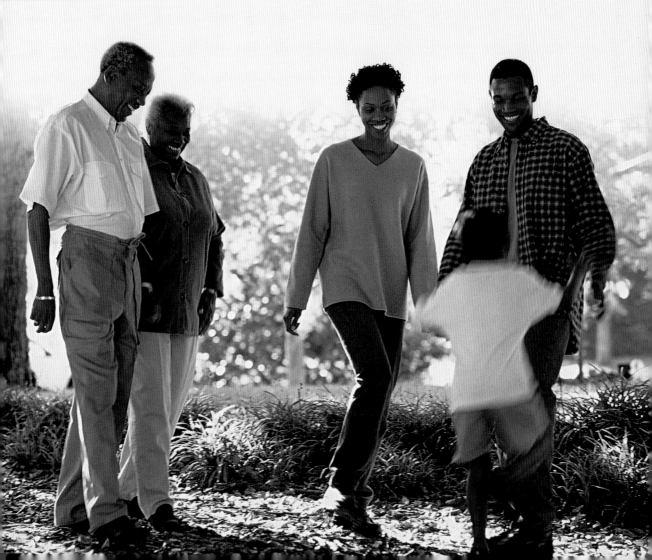

Your joints

Joints are the places where our bones meet and move. They allow us to bend and twist, to jump, swim, run, to play a piano, pick up a pin and kick a football around in the park. But when we get arthritis, joints can be the source of misery.

There are three kind of joints. Those called the *synarthroses*, such as the bones in the skull, have little or no movement and are not affected by arthritis.

The *amphiarthroses* are joints with some movement. They hold together our pelvis, and make up the spinal column. In the spine, cartilage disks are sandwiched between the vertebrae to allow us to bend and twist. Arthritis can develop in these joints, especially in the neck (cervical) or lower back (lumbar) vertebrae.

The joints most vulnerable to arthritis are called *diarthroses*, or synovial joints. These are the very mobile joints in our knees, hips, shoulders, arms, legs and knuckles of our fingers. Synovial joints are enclosed in a joint capsule which is made up of tough fibres and lined with a thin layer of membrane called the synovium. This membrane secretes a slippery fluid called synovial fluid that lubricates and nourishes the internal part of the joint.

Covering the ends of the bones in each joint is a layer of cartilage. This tough, spongy material acts as a shock absorber and provides a smooth gliding surface for joint motion. Your knees have another fibrous cartilage pad called a *meniscus*, which acts like a cushion between the two parts of the knee joint.

The entire joint capsule is held in place by a complex array of ligaments, muscles and tendons that attach to the capsule and the bones above and below the joint, and help it to move.

WARNING SIGNS TO SEE YOUR DOCTOR

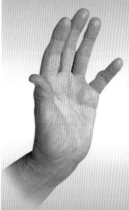

Some kinds of arthritis need early and aggressive treatment to prevent or lessen irreversible joint damage. Infectious arthritis, for example, can be cured when treated with antibiotics – if you think you might have an infection, call your doctor at once. Joint damage from rheumatoid arthritis can be reduced or prevented with powerful drugs. If you notice any of the following, see your doctor:

* Constant or recurring pain or tenderness in a joint that lasts for more than two weeks.
* Swelling in one or more joints, especially with warmth and redness.
* Stiffness around the joints that lasts for at least an hour in the early morning.
* Sudden difficulty using or moving a joint normally.

Maintaining healthy joints

Joints and the tissues around them can be damaged by injuries, infection and many kinds of arthritis. It is important to avoid joint injuries if you can, or treat them promptly, since arthritis is more likely to develop in joints that have been injured.

Muscle, ligament and tendon sprains and strains should also be treated promptly, since they are essential to keep your joints in line. Sometimes you may need surgery. Most kinds of arthritis cannot be cured yet, but there is plenty you can do to ease pain and inflammation, and to keep these symptoms from getting worse.

Joints were made to be moved – even joints with arthritis. Exercise is essential to maintain mobility. When you flex your joints, you are helping to keep them healthy by keeping the supporting muscles strong and pumping fluids through the cartilage lining. But do be careful: inappropriate exercise can aggravate an inflammatory condition, so consult your doctor if you have arthritis.

Doctors also advise maintaining the appropriate weight for your age and body type. Excess weight stresses joints – even those of your hands. Flat, supportive shoes help to relieve stress on knees and hips by keeping your gait balanced and legs aligned properly. A balanced diet rich in vegetables and low in meat and saturated fats gives your body fuel to maintain healthy joints. Conventional and complementary medicine offer ways to ease pain and sometimes stop joint breakdown.

WHAT CAUSES ARTHRITIS?

Researchers don't know yet what causes most of the many different kinds of arthritis that attack the joints and connective tissues. However, risk factors for some kinds of arthritis include:

- **Being a woman** Some types of arthritis, such as lupus, rheumatoid arthritis and fibromyalgia, affect primarily women. Overall, nearly twice as many women as men get arthritis.
- **Being a man** Ankylosing spondylitis and gout primarily affect men.
- **Heredity** A tendency towards some types of arthritis may be inherited, including susceptibility to autoimmune diseases and a weakness in joints or bones that makes you more at risk from injury.
- **Repeated joint injuries or stresses** Sports or work activities can damage or even wear away cartilage in the joints.
- **Obesity** Being overweight puts extra stress on knees and hips, and can contribute to osteoarthritis and gout.

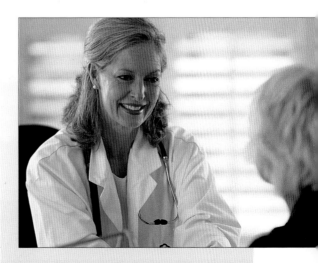

Osteoarthritis (OA)

Sometimes called degenerative joint disease, OA results when the cushioning cartilage in joints breaks down or wears away, causing pain and stiffness.

OA is the most common form of arthritis, affecting most people to some degree after the age of 60. But the severity varies greatly: some people have only mild aches and some stiffness while others may be disabled. Pain is the main symptom and even that varies – some people with severe OA have little or no pain.

What happens?

Cartilage is the gristle in our joints that cushions the bone endings and helps joints to move smoothly. As we age, cartilage begins to lose its flexibility and becomes more vulnerable to damage from overuse or injuries. It begins to actually wear away, putting the joints under stress, which in turn speeds up cartilage destruction. This causes bones to thicken or change shape, and narrows the space within a joint,

---

RISK FACTORS

Some conditions can make your OA worse or increase your risk of getting it at a younger age:

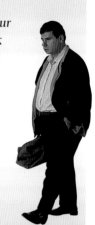

- Being overweight, which puts stress on joints.
- Repeated injuries or stress to joints.
- Stress on a joint due to its repeated use.
- Heredity.
- Weakened muscles that don't support the joints.

---

causing pain (*see box, page 17*). In severe cases, all of the cushioning cartilage may be destroyed, leaving bones in direct contact with no "padding", causing more pain and limiting movement in that joint.

OA usually affects just a few joints. It most commonly affects the knees, hips, hands, neck and lower spine. OA may also show up in the joint of your big toe as a bunion or as bony spurs on your fingers – those appearing at the end joints of the fingers are called Heberden's nodes; those at the middle joints are Bouchard's nodes.

Diagnosing OA

OA is usually diagnosed by examining your joints and listening to you describe your symptoms. Laboratory tests might rule out other joint conditions that would need aggressive treatment, such as infectious or rheumatoid arthritis. OA can be seen on

---

SYMPTOMS OF OA

- Pain in a joint that increases with use and that is relieved when you rest.
- Stiffness and a decreased range of motion.
- Gradual enlargement of the joints.
- Crackling or grating sounds when you move your joints.
- Sometimes, swelling and inflammation in the joint.

X-rays and other imaging tests. The X-ray will show a narrowing of the joint spaces, the presence of bone spurs or damage to bone surfaces inside the joints.

Treatment of OA

The main goals of treatment are pain relief, protecting joints from more damage and helping you stay active. Top priorities are keeping a proper weight and exercising daily. Often, pain can be eased with non-prescription drugs, such as paracetamol, and non-steroidal anti-inflammatory drugs (NSAIDs), such as ibuprofen and aspirin (*see page 53*). If you take these medicines, follow the instructions on the pack and ask your doctor's advice as most NSAIDs can cause stomach ulcers.

If there is inflammation, more powerful NSAIDs may be ordered. Braces, supportive shoes or inserts (orthodics) and using a cane may help ease stress on knees, feet and hips with arthritis. Injections of hyaluronic acid can bring temporary relief. Surgery, such as joint replacement (*see page 61*), can restore movement in cases of severe cartilage loss.

AN OSTEOARTHRITIC JOINT

When joints move, the cartilage that lines the ends of the bones absorbs the shock and prevents damage to the bones. The cartilage is elastic and very slick, allowing bones to slide over one another smoothly. In OA, the cartilage of the joint is damaged and wearing away or else it has degenerated entirely.

Researchers are still investigating causes of cartilage destruction, looking at chemical processes that lead to inflammation in the joint. Injuries or stress from being overweight can hasten that process by damaging cartilage. Lack of exercise contributes as the cartilage has no blood supply of its own and depends on joint movement to pump nutrients through its tissues.

In OA, the cartilage loses the ability to repair itself. It becomes thinner and less able to absorb nutrients. Eventually it begins to fray, split and wear away. Bones that had been protected by shock-absorbing cartilage become exposed and then rub against each other, causing more damage. The bone ends thicken, forming bony spurs, or osteophytes, and the joint becomes stiff and painful.

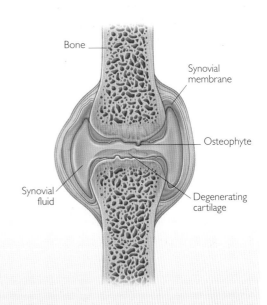

Bone

Synovial membrane

Osteophyte

Synovial fluid

Degenerating cartilage

Rheumatoid arthritis (RA)

One of the most serious and disabling types of arthritis, RA is believed to be an autoimmune disease, which means that the body's immune system mistakenly attacks its own healthy tissue (*see box, page 19*). An infection could trigger RA, and hormones may play a role, since it strikes three times as many women as men. It can also be life-threatening.

In RA, the immune system attacks the synovium (joint lining) and may also attack internal organs, resulting in pain, inflammation and, in some cases, joint deformity (*see box, page 19*). It usually begins in the young- to middle-adult years, but can attack young children or infants.

What happens?

RA may make you run a fever and ache all over your body. You may also become anaemic and have dryness of the eyes and mouth caused by the inflammation of the tear ducts and the salivary glands. RA can also cause inflammation in the lungs, blood vessels and nerves.

RISK FACTORS

It is not known why some people's immune systems become destructive, but your risk increases if:

- You are female. Three times more women than men get RA.
- Others in your family have autoimmune diseases.
- You are a smoker. Women who smoke for more than 20 years have up to 39 per cent higher risk of getting RA.

SYMPTOMS OF RA

- Swelling, pain, warmth, redness and soreness in the joints.
- Pain or stiffness on awakening that lasts more than an hour.
- Swelling or pain in several joints on both sides of the body.
- Sometimes fever and enlarged lymph nodes.

It can be frustrating and depressing to cope with RA because it is so unpredictable and so painful. Symptoms can come and go without warning and vary from person to person. Some have an initial flare of RA, and then go for months or years without further attacks. But most people suffer through cycles of flares and remissions. A small percentage may have severe symptoms that worsen with no remissions.

RA is a serious disease. Untreated, it can take years off a person's life, so early and aggressive treatment for all types of RA is crucial to prevent or slow down joint damage and keep you active. Many with RA, especially older people, also have OA.

Diagnosing RA

No single test can diagnose RA, but a variety of examinations can rule out other diseases. Your doctor will take your medical history, asking if others in your family have had RA, and order laboratory tests to look at levels of rheumatoid factor (an antibody in the blood) and measure erythrocyte sedimentation rate (ESR) which shows the level of inflammation. You may need X-rays, bone scans or other imaging tests, or a biopsy of fluid or tissue from your joint.

Treatment of RA

Doctors focus on getting inflammation under control to prevent permanent joint damage (*see Chapter Three*). Non-steroidal anti-inflammatory drugs (NSAIDs) may work in mild cases. In more severe cases, doctors may turn to corticosteroids, such as prednisolone in pills, or injections.

There are many powerful disease-modifying anti-rheumatic drugs (DMARDs) to slow or halt inflammation, including hydroxychloroquine sulphate, methotrexate, leflunomide and azathioprine. In addition, there is a whole new class of drugs called biologic response modifiers (BRMs), which include imfliximab and etanercept. Doctors also recommend taking regular exercise,

A RHEUMATOID ARTHRITIC JOINT

Rheumatoid arthritis attacks the lining (synovium) of the joint, causing the membrane to become inflamed and swollen. RA affects the same joints on both sides of the body, usually the joints of the hands and feet but it may also affect the hips, knees and other joints.

White blood cells are part of the immune system, the body's defence against bacteria, viruses and other diseases. In RA, it is thought that these cells mistakenly attack the body they are meant to protect. They move into the joint tissues and fluid accumulates that produces substances, such as enzymes, antibodies and cytokines, that mistakenly attack the lining of the joint and other joint tissues.

The accumulated fluid causes the joint to swell and the joint capsule becomes deformed and painful. The continued inflammation can be very destructive, damaging cartilage, bone, tendons and ligaments. Joints severely affected by RA become weak and unstable, and may be permanently damaged if inflammation is not controlled. These joints may become deformed, causing disability.

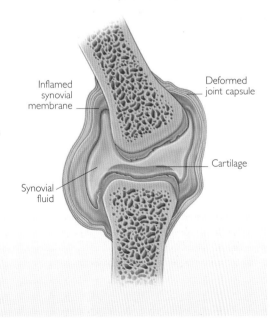

Inflamed synovial membrane

Synovial fluid

Deformed joint capsule

Cartilage

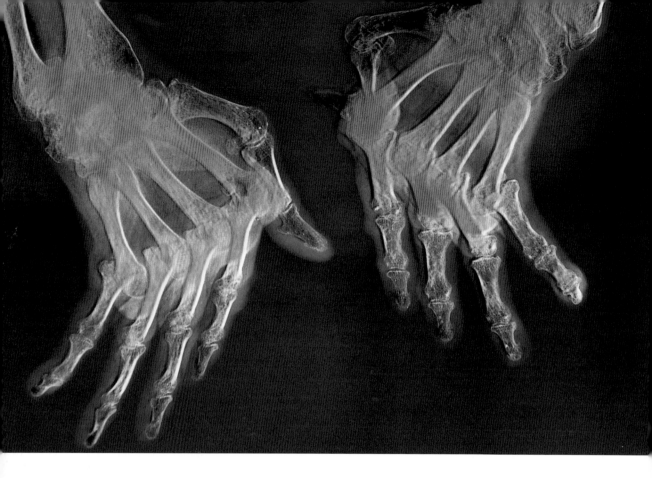

applying pain–easing ointments (*see page 52*), and, if necessary, undergoing joint surgery or joint replacement (*see page 61*).

Juvenile idiopathic arthritis

Babies and young children are not immune to many types of arthritis. Most common is juvenile idiopathic arthritis, also called juvenile rheumatoid arthritis, which can be mild or very severe. It generally follows the same pattern of symptoms as in adult RA. Juvenile idiopathic arthritis can be very difficult to diagnose, since some symptoms resemble other childhood diseases.

The least common form, called systemic onset juvenile rheumatoid arthritis, can be the most severe. It attacks the entire body, usually includes high fever (103° F/39.4° C

X-RAY OF HANDS SHOWING RHEUMATOID ARTHRITIS
This false-colour X-ray of the hands of a person suffering from extreme rheumatoid arthritis shows just how devastating the disease can be. The joints of all the fingers in both hands have been affected.

or more), a rash, joint inflammation and deformities. It can cause inflammation of the lining of the heart or lungs, and enlargement of the lymph nodes, liver or spleen. If not treated aggressively and early, juvenile idiopathic arthritis can cause joint deformities and disability.

Other forms of arthritis which attack children include juvenile spondylo–arthropathies (*see also Ankylosing spondylitis, page 23*), which are diseases of the spine, and forms of lupus, psoriatic arthritis and scleroderma (*see page 23*).

Fibromyalgia

Fibromyalgia is a chronic pain syndrome related to arthritis that affects the fibrous connective tissue and muscles. It can be disabling and often accompanies other types of arthritis, particularly RA and systemic lupus. Fibromyalgia affects mostly women, causing fatigue, sleep disturbances, depression and widespread pain in muscles and tendons, particularly in the neck, spine, shoulders and hips. While it is not life-threatening, the extreme fatigue and pain can lead to disability and muscle weakness from lack of activity.

What happens?

Fibromyalgia pain is not in the joints, but in the muscles, ligaments and tendons. It may be triggered by an infection, a physical trauma from an accident or surgery, or an emotional trauma from physical, sexual or other abuse. It is also connected with abnormal levels of substance P, which transports pain messages; a growth hormone called somatomedin C; or the hormone serotonin, which helps regulate sleep, mood and pain perception.

SYMPTOMS OF FIBROMYALGIA

* Pain in 11 of 18 specific tender points.
* Muscle aches all over the body.
* Fatigue.
* Insomnia or other sleep disorders.
* Depression and anxiety.
* Irritable bowel syndrome.
* Tension headache and migraine headache.

RISK FACTORS

* Being a woman.
* Injury, trauma or major surgery.
* Physical, sexual or emotional abuse.
* Stress.
* Sleep deprivation.

Diagnosing fibromyalgia

Difficult to diagnose, fibromyalgia was once mistaken for fibrositis and is often confused with chronic fatigue syndrome.

People with fibromyalgia often do not look sick or show abnormalities in laboratory tests but say they have almost constant and sometimes terrible pain. Their doctor may order tests to rule out other conditions and base the diagnosis on pain in at least 11 of 18 specific tender point sites.

Treatment of fibromyalgia

It is difficult to treat fibromyalgia since the symptoms can vary so widely and the cause is unknown. Doctors usually concentrate on trying to relieve pain and help with sleep, prescribing analgesics, such as paracetamol, and even more powerful pain medications.

Low doses of antidepressants and muscle relaxants may help with sleep and mood. Meditation, visualization and other mind body practices, such as tai chi and qigong, have been found to ease some symptoms – sometimes dramatically. Exercise also helps, although it might be the last thing you feel like doing if you're in a lot of pain.

Gout & other types of arthritis

Gout pain is excruciating and unmistakable. It's caused by high blood levels of uric acid, a substance produced by the breakdown of purines in alcohol and foods such as lentils, dried beans, anchovies, sardines, shellfish and organ meats, such as kidney and liver.

The first attack comes without warning, and often in bed at night and usually in the big toe. The first few attacks fade after a few days. Untreated, the episodes are more frequent, last longer, attack more joints and may cause permanent damage.

What happens?

Rich foods have high levels of purines, which the body breaks down into uric acid and other chemicals. These are normally eliminated through the kidneys in urine. But in people with gout, that system goes awry: uric acid builds up in the blood, forming sharp crystals that collect in the joints and soft tissues, causing inflammation and sometimes agonizing pain.

RISK FACTORS

- Being a middle-aged man or a post-menopausal woman.
- Being overweight.
- Consuming large amounts of alcohol and foods with purines, such as red meats and shellfish.
- Heredity.

SYMPTOMS OF GOUT

- Severe pain in one joint (often the big toe).
- Swelling, redness, warmth and extreme tenderness of the joint.
- Fever, chills, fatigue and loss of appetite.

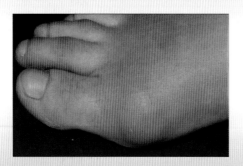

Gout often starts in the big toe when crystals of uric acid accumulate in the joint capsule. These cause the joint to become swollen and purplish-red.

Diagnosing gout

Laboratory tests include checking for uric acid levels, and examining your joints and soft tissue for uric acid deposits. If gout is advanced, X-rays or other imaging tests can determine joint damage. Your doctor will check your other medications as some drugs can contribute to high uric acid levels.

Treatment of gout

Getting the inflammation down is a priority. NSAIDs may help. Powerful medications to control gout include colchicine, allopurinol and corticosteroids.

You may greatly reduce or even stop future attacks by carefully changing your diet to avoid purines and alcohol, losing weight and exercising.

OTHER TYPES OF ARTHRITIS AND RELATED CONDITIONS

As well osteoarthritis, rheumatoid arthritis, fibromyalgia and gout there are many less common kinds of arthritis and musculoskeletal conditions that can affect the joints in the body. The following are some of the more than 100 kinds of arthritis:

LUPUS

Systemic lupus erythematosus (SLE) is a serious autoimmune disorder affecting mostly women. It can inflame and damage joints, connective tissues and internal organs, and may cause inflammation of the lining of the heart and lungs, and kidney and blood problems.

ANKYLOSING SPONDYLITIS

This type of arthritis usually attacks the spine, but may also cause arthritis in the shoulders, hips and knees. In severe cases, the vertebrae "freeze" together. Mostly, it appears to attack men in late adolescence or early adulthood, and seems to be inherited.

INFECTIOUS ARTHRITIS

Bacterial or viral infections can cause joints to inflame and, left untreated, can cause permanent damage. If treated early, most bacterial types can be cured with antibiotics. If a joint or joints become painful and inflamed fairly quickly, you should consult your doctor at once.

PSORIATIC ARTHRITIS

About 10 per cent of people with psoriasis also develop a form of inflammatory arthritis. Inflammation can occur in the synovium and where tendons attach to bones, particularly at the ends of the fingers and toes and in the lower back.

POLYMYALGIA RHEUMATICA

This is a rheumatic disease affecting tendons, muscles, ligaments and tissues around the joints. It can cause pain, aching and morning stiffness in the neck, shoulders, lower back and hips, and usually responds dramatically to medical treatment. Giant cell arteritis (a disease of the arteries characterized by inflammation, weakness, weight loss and fever) is more common in people with polymyalgia.

RAYNAUD'S PHENOMENON

This results when blood vessels in the hands and feet spasm, temporarily restricting blood circulation. It can sometimes lead to skin ulcers. Raynaud's phenomenon affects mainly women and it often occurs along with scleroderma and lupus. Treatment includes keeping warm, protecting the skin and, sometimes, drugs to reduce spasms and help circulation.

SCLERODERMA

This serious disease (also known as systemic sclerosis) is due to an overproduction of collagen (a fibre-like protein) that makes tissues stiff and hard – the word scleroderma means "hard skin". It can be deadly: it affects the skin, blood vessels and joints, and, in a more serious form, attacks internal organs, such as the lungs and kidneys. It affects mostly women between the ages of 30 and 50.

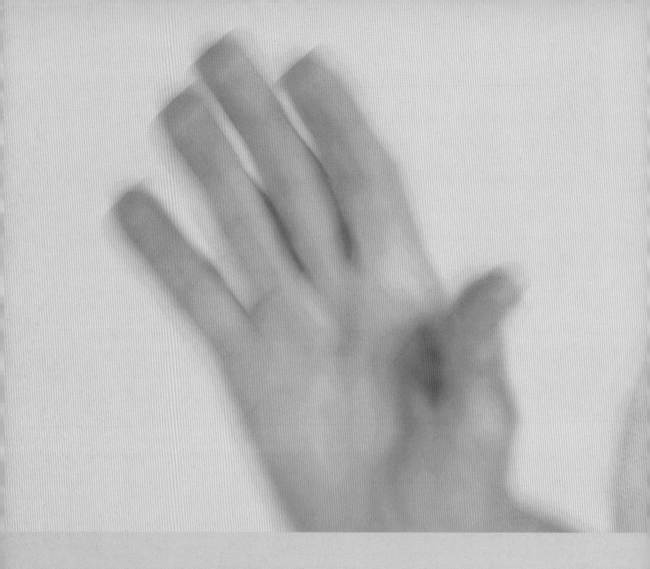

Self-help for
arthritis

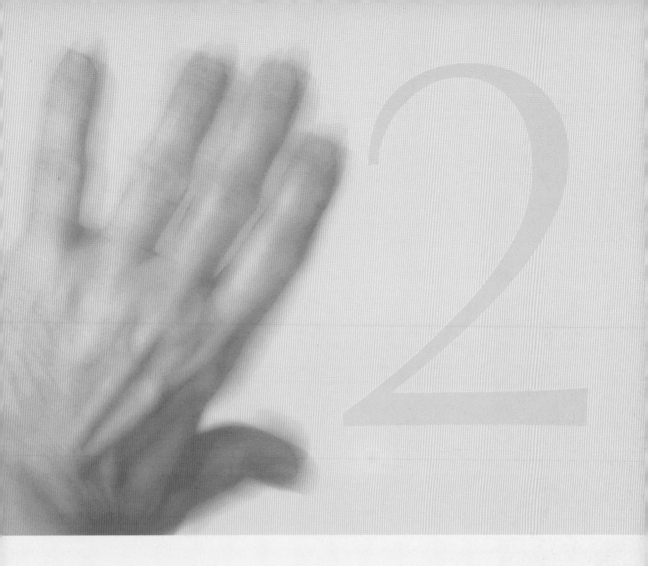

People who take an active and positive role in the treatment of their illness feel better and do better, no matter what kind of arthritis they have. They tend to have less pain and more energy, and to stay active and independent.

A healthy diet

There are thousands of books and articles that talk about special diets for just about everything, including arthritis. So far, there are no foods proven to cause arthritis and no special diets that can "cure" your arthritis. A good "arthritis diet" is one that helps you to maintain a weight appropriate for your age and body type, offsets the effects of your arthritis medication and improves your overall health.

Being overweight greatly increases your risks of developing arthritis and of making it worse – in particular osteoarthritis of the knees. You'll also increase your risk of developing other diseases, such as adult onset diabetes and heart disease. Being underweight is bad for your health, too. People with rheumatoid arthritis quite often are too thin – perhaps the pain and disability prevent shopping, interfere with cooking or decrease the appetite.

Weight issues can contribute to your arthritis symptoms by keeping you from exercising. It's a vicious circle. If you are overweight, it may hurt to exercise. If you are underweight, you may be too tired. But if you don't exercise, your joints become more at risk from arthritis.

Adjusting your diet

The very medications that help your arthritis can deplete your body of vital nutrients so it's important to eat nutritious foods and, if necessary, take dietary supplements. A daily multivitamin may be all you need, but you may need to take extra vitamins or minerals.

Food allergies that could contribute to arthritis are rare, but a sensitivity to certain foods may make symptoms worse. So keep a food journal for several weeks, noting what you eat and if any particular food seems to make your symptoms worse, then stop eating it. Fasting may also help some symptoms but it isn't a long-term solution. Fad diets or very restrictive diets don't seem to help and may even harm your health.

Overall, nutrition experts recommend a balanced diet: high in vegetables and fruits with plenty of fibre and fresh water, and low in saturated fats and meat. Studies show that some people with rheumatoid arthritis have improved on a vegetarian diet. Eliminating fried foods, sweets and snack foods can also help you to maintain a proper weight.

A healthy diet goes beyond what you eat. It involves changes in the way you shop, cook and even think about food, and it goes on forever. It may take a big effort to overcome old eating habits. But the rewards are worth it. You will have better joint health, and will feel and look better.

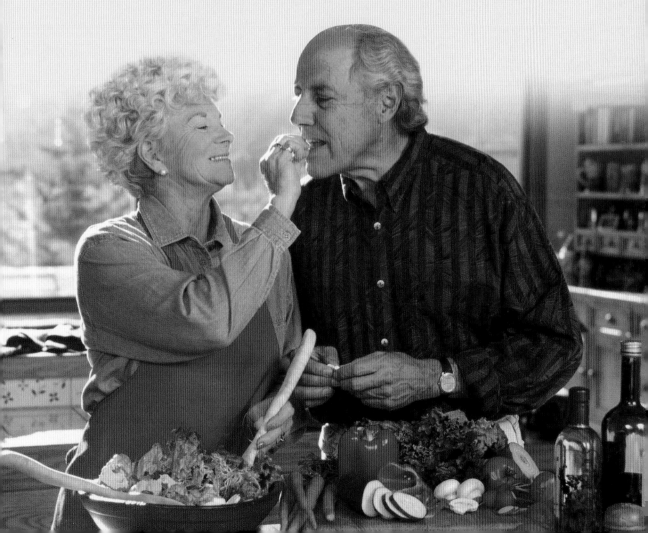

Healing foods

Some foods are especially important for people with arthritis because they contain ingredients that replace valuable nutrients lost through certain arthritis medications. Research reveals that particular foods can help ease inflammation or pain and that others may contribute to symptoms.

Antioxidants

Our cells can be damaged by substances called "free radicals" – destructive molecules circulating in our blood and in our cells. Free radicals help to defend us against bacteria, but too many can cause trouble by damaging cells and increasing disease risks.

Antioxidants can help to prevent this damage. They include betacarotene (a vegetable form of vitamin A) and vitamins C and E. But before you rush to buy these as supplements, consider changing your diet and start eating five portions of fruit and vegetables daily. A diet high in natural antioxidants is best for your overall health and for maintaining a good weight. An added benefit is that the foods may have more than one antioxidant.

The highest levels of betacarotene are to be found in bright orange carrots and sweet potatoes. Many fruits and vegetables contain vitamin C: whole, fresh fruits and vegetables are the best source of vitamins. In particular, eat cruciferous vegetables (*see page 29*), such as broccoli, and dark, leafy greens. Vitamin E is found in grains, beans, nuts and many fruits and vegetables.

Chilli pepper

Capsaicin, the ingredient that makes red peppers hot, can help ease joint pain when applied externally in creams and ointments. It works by interfering with the actions of a pain transmitter known as substance P.

The ointment may irritate your skin at first. Take care not to get any in or near your eyes or other sensitive areas. It can give substantial – but temporary – relief and is best used when only one or two joints are involved, as in OA.

FOODS IN AN OINTMENT
Rubbing a cream or ointment made from chilli pepper into a painful joint, such as the knee, can bring you temporary relief from pain.

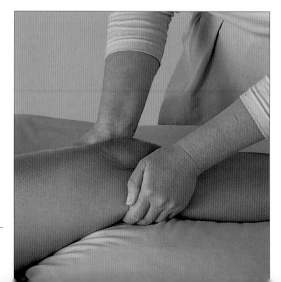

Copper-rich foods

Copper deficiency may be connected with arthritis but it is rare, and copper pill supplements have not been studied. If you suspect you have low copper levels, try copper-rich foods, such as nuts, barley and wheat germ – and chocolate, crab, lobster, oysters and red wine. But remember: these are not all good for you if you have gout and they may contribute to high cholesterol. Copper bracelets have long been a "therapy" for arthritis but there is no scientific evidence they have any effect.

Cruciferous vegetables

These dark green vegetables, named after the cross shape in their flowers, are among the best foods for general health. They contain vitamins and minerals known to reduce the risks of developing arthritis – and they also help to reduce risks of cancer and heart disease. They include broccoli, Brussels sprouts, spinach, bok choy, the cabbages, collard greens and kale. Consider them as a treasure chest as they contain antioxidant vitamins A, C and E as well as boron, calcium, magnesium and selenium. And they are low in calories.

Flaxseed

Flaxseed is the richest plant source of the constituents of omega-3 oils (*see page 30*), which have been shown to help relieve inflammation. You can use flaxseed as a meal in baking and make a salad dressing with the oil. Only cook with the oil under low heat as too much will damage it.

Fish

Cold-water, oily fish, such as mackerel, tuna, salmon, herring and sardines, are high in omega-3 oils (*see page 30*), which help to reduce inflammation and are good for heart health. The fish also contain vitamins D, E and B12 along with calcium. Eat oily fish every week. **Caution:** if you are pregnant or breastfeeding beware of fish from areas high in mercury.

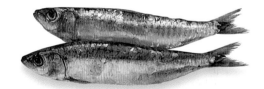

Ginger

The root of the ginger lily, this tangy spice is used in cooking throughout Asia. It is also a popular remedy for nausea, indigestion and arthritis. It can be grated fresh to make tea or used in sauces, condiments, stir fries, cakes and sweets.

Ginger contains substances that are said to inhibit the production of prostaglandins and leukotrienes which trigger inflammation and pain. Studies of a combination product showed that it eased pain and swelling for both OA and RA.

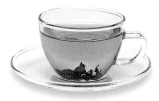

Green tea

An everyday drink in Asia, green tea is high in polyphenols and is believed to help prevent cancer. Animal studies suggest green tea may also help to relieve arthritis inflammation. Green tea contains caffeine so you can drink it instead of coffee, which may contribute to RA.

Omega–3 oils

Researchers are showing that the kind of oils you eat can affect your health. They do not suggest that you cut out all oils: in fact, they say adding some oils to your diet and cutting back on others might help reduce arthritis inflammation.

We need essential fatty acids from a variety of sources. But our modern diets, which contain processed and convenience foods, are out of balance. We tend to get too many "bad" animal fats, saturated fats and vegetable fats containing omega–6 linoleic fatty acids that may contribute to inflammation. And we do not consume enough foods that contain "good" omega–3 linolenic fatty acids.

Nutritionists suggest that we can get our oils back in balance by cutting back on foods full of linoleic acids, such as meat, most processed and fast foods, and most cooking oils. Instead, consider replacing these foods with those that are high in omega–3 fatty acids, such as cold–water oily fish (*see page 29*), and flaxseed (*see page 29*), rapeseed and olive oils.

Supplements may also help: in some studies, people with RA who took fish oil supplements were able to significantly reduce their use of NSAIDs. There is also promising research that shows gamma–linolenic acid (GLA) supplements (*see page 72*) can reduce inflammation.

ALLERGIES AND SENSITIVITIES

True food allergies are rare. But researchers are finding that some people are sensitive to certain foods, which may make their arthritis symptoms worse or even trigger a flare (when symptoms suddenly get worse). The response is very specific: there is no list of foods to which everyone with arthritis reacts. Some of the foods known to trigger symptoms are listed below.

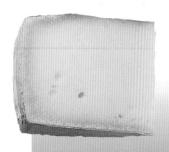

FOODS THAT MIGHT TRIGGER A FLARE

- MILK, CHEESE AND OTHER DAIRY PRODUCTS ● CORN PRODUCTS
- WHEAT PRODUCTS ● MEAT (ESPECIALLY COLD CUTS AND PRESERVED MEATS)
- EGGS ● CITRUS FRUITS – ORANGES, GRAPEFRUITS, LEMONS ● TOMATOES
- PEANUTS ● COFFEE ● SOY

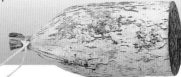
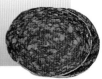

Organic foods

Foods grown and processed without using chemical fertilizers, pesticides, hormones or other man–made additives are increasingly easy to find. Eating organic may help, as these foods don't contain chemicals that might provoke a reaction and contribute to arthritis symptoms.

Tomatoes

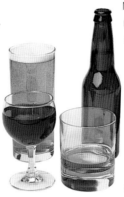

Many people believe that food derived from the nightshade family – tomatoes, potatoes and aubergines – can increase arthritis symptoms. The promoter of the idea, a horticulturist named Norman Childers, collected the statements of thousands of people who reported an improvement in the symptoms of their arthritis when they avoided foods from the nightshade family. But this has not been studied in a scientifically accepted manner. Tomatoes, in fact, are a helpful food: a rich source of vitamins, antioxidants and lycopenes, which are known to reduce cancer risks. But if tomatoes seem to bother your arthritis, then don't eat them.

Turmeric

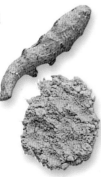

Used liberally in curries and sauces, this is an ancient Ayurvedic treatment for arthritis. Studies show it has anti–inflammatory chemicals and, used with other spices, turmeric has been shown to relieve both OA and RA pain.

DRINKS THAT HURT HEALTH

Some drinks are not good for people with arthritis. Consider consuming the following in moderation or removing them from your diet altogether.

ALCOHOL DRINKS

You may have heard a glass of wine a day is good for heart health. No-one with arthritis should have more than two glasses per day and some people with arthritis should not drink at all. Remember that alcohol can be dangerous when taken with some arthritis medications, including paracetamol, NSAIDs (see page 53) and methotrexate. It contains chemicals that may increase uric acid levels and contribute to gout (see page 22). Alcohol consumption also contributes to bone density loss, and adds "empty" extra calories that can contribute to weight gain.

COFFEE DRINKS

Many people with fibromyalgia who have irritable bowel syndrome will find their condition improves without coffee. Coffee may also contribute to the risk of developing RA. One Finnish study found that people who drank more than three cups a day had twice the chance of getting the disease as those who drank less. Another study looked at middle-aged women of Nordic descent in the American Midwest and found those who drank more than 2.5 cups of decaffeinated coffee a day have double the risk of developing adult onset RA.

Dietary supplements

"Miracle cures" for arthritis in pills, potions and lotions are advertised everywhere, often with extravagant claims and glowing testimonials. Few of these are backed with any scientific proof. Most are useless and some may even be dangerous. In fact, the more outrageous the claim, the more likely the product is to be useless.

However, mixed among the many fake "cures" are some dietary supplements that may help ease the pain and inflammation of arthritis. Here is an overview of some of the most popular dietary supplements.

Glucosamine and chondroitin

If you have osteoarthritis, you've probably heard about glucosamine and chondroitin. These two supplements are well–publicized for easing the pain and stiffness of OA, and

A WORD OF WARNING

Don't give up or reduce the dosage of your prescription drugs without consulting your doctor. Be aware that supplements may have side effects or interact with your drugs. Tell your doctor what you 're taking and of any unusual symptoms. Follow the instructions on the pack and if the supplement doesn't seem to work after a month or so, stop taking it.

may even help repair or rebuild cartilage. Doctors generally agree these supplements are safe and may help your symptoms.

Both glucosamine and chondroitin have been studied and used across Europe and Asia for more than two decades and are prescription drugs in several countries.

SUPPLEMENTS OF QUESTIONABLE VALUE

Remarkable claims have been made for many supplements but until scientific research shows them to be effective and safe, it is best not to try them. Here are two examples:

GREEN-LIPPED MUSSELS

This remedy from New Zealand has been widely touted for RA. But results from the one study that showed it to be effective have not been confirmed. The remedy may be contaminated – one case of hepatitis was reported – and it may provoke seafood or shellfish allergic reactions. Not recommended.

METHYL SULPHONYL METHANE (MSM)

This product is supposed to ease pain and inflammation from just about anything. It is a sulphur compound and probably not harmful, but there are no human studies to show if it is effective or safe. Pills, capsules, creams, lotions and crystalline bath salts are available.

Glucosamine – in both its hydrochloride (HCL) and sulphate forms – comes from the chitin in the shell of shellfish and lobsters. Chondroitin sulphate comes from the trachea (windpipe) of cattle. Both appear to slow or stop OA by nourishing the cartilage and by blocking inflammation and the enzymes that break down cartilage.

Numerous studies on thousands of people have shown both glucosamine and chondroitin relieve OA pain about as well NSAIDs, such as ibuprofen, naproxen and aspirin, but without the dangerous gastrointestinal and other side effects.

They may also help to repair or rebuild cartilage, according to two studies. In the glucosamine study, 1,500mg of glucosamine was given daily in a drink to 106 people with OA of the knee. After three years, X–rays of their knees showed, on average, none of the joint space narrowing that is indicative of OA progression.

The chondroitin study showed that patients with OA of the finger joints, who took 1,200mg of chondroitin daily for three years, had less joint erosion than those who took a placebo (a sugar pill).

That's exciting news. But these supplements may not work for everyone. Studies suggest they will not help your symptoms if your OA is very severe; if you have little or no cartilage

S-ADENOSYLMETHIONINE (SAMe)

SAMe is a naturally occurring compound in all living cells. It is a key player in a process called methlyation that affects more than 100 complex biochemical reactions in the human body.

SAMe is known to ease both OA pain and depression, and to have few or no side effects or interactions with other medications. Doctors in Europe have studied and used SAMe for more than two decades and it's a prescription drug in several countries.

Controlled clinical trials show that SAMe relieves OA pain as well as NSAIDs, such as ibuprofen. The trials also show that it eases fibromyalgia symptoms for some people.

SAMe works as well as tricyclic anti-depressants in improving mood, and there is also evidence that it may help repair liver damage. However, there's no evidence that SAMe helps to repair cartilage.

People with bi-polar disease (manic depression) or serious emotional problems should not take SAMe without a doctor's supervision. Also, SAMe is not very stable – it disintegrates quickly so some supplements may not have any active ingredients – and it's expensive. Look for products with packaging that protects them from heat and light.

Usual dose: in tablets. For OA, 200 to 400mg three times per day. For fibromyalgia, 200mg per day to begin with, then increasing to 800mg per day. For depression, consult your doctor.

remaining in your joints; or if you are very overweight. You may have to take these supplements for several months before you notice any effect and you have to continue to take them every day.

There is no evidence that one of these supplements is better than the other at relieving OA symptoms or that they are better taken in combination than alone. A major study in the USA involving more than 1,000 people with arthritis is presently underway, but the results are not due to published for several years.

Both supplements are available as pills, capsules or chewables, or as crystals for a ready-to-mix drink. Usual dosage per day: 1,500mg of glucosamine (either sulphate or HCL form); 1,200mg of chondroitin.

Vitamins and minerals

These basics are essential for good health, and eating a balanced diet with plenty of fresh fruit and vegetables will usually provide you with adequate supplies.

However, this may not be possible for some people; shopping and preparing food may be difficult due to pain. Also, the effects of medication or inflammation can result in poor nutrient absorption.

Usually, a multivitamin supplement will ensure you get all the necessary nutrients. You may need extra amounts of some – but there is no evidence that megadoses of a particular vitamin or mineral help arthritis. Too much of some supplements can be dangerous while others may block or interfere with your prescription drugs.

MINERALS

A balanced diet or a multivitamin usually provides all the minerals we need. Supplements may help with some symptoms. Do not exceed the suggested dosages without consulting your doctor.

CALCIUM

All women past menopause and all people with arthritis need extra calcium, from supplements or diet, especially those taking corticosteroids. Usual dose: 1,000 to 1,200mg per day.

MAGNESIUM

Supplements of magnesium, combined with malic acid, ease pain associated with fibromyalgia. Check with your doctor, as it may interact with other drugs. High doses have a laxative effect. Usual dose: 1,200–2,400mg malic acid with 300–600mg magnesium taken daily.

SELENIUM

People with inflammatory types of arthritis may have low selenium levels. Supplements ease tenderness, stiffness and swelling. You may get the little you need in a multivitamin. Usual dose: 50–200 micrograms per day.

ZINC

Most popular as a cold cure, studies show zinc might ease symptoms of RA and psoriatic arthritis. We only need a little and too much could affect your "good" cholesterol balance. Check with a doctor for the best dosage.

VITAMINS

Vitamins are essential for health and well-being and are best taken from a diet rich in vegetables, grains and fruits. Extra vitamins may help offset the effects of some kinds of arthritis – or the medications we take for them. Do not exceed the suggested dosages without consulting your doctor first. More is not necessarily better and may, in fact, be harmful.

VITAMIN B3 (NIACIN)

One study found B3 supplements increase the effectiveness of NSAIDs in relieving pain and stiffness associated with OA and RA. Vitamin B3 may interfere with diabetes drugs. Usual dose: 10–25mg per day.

VITAMIN B5 (PANTOTHENIC ACID)

There is some evidence that vitamin B5 levels may be low in people with RA and that B5 supplements helped with the morning stiffness and pain associated with RA. Usual dose: 250mg per day.

FOLIC ACID

Doctors recommend that people taking methotrexate (*see page 54*) also take a folic acid (folate) supplement to offset possible drug side effects. It is also recommended for people with lupus, who may have higher homocysteine levels associated with stroke and heart disease. Many foods are fortified with folic acid as well. Usual dose: 1mg per day. For lupus, this dose is taken with 5mg of B6 vitamin and 1mg of B12 vitamin.

VITAMIN C

Megadoses of vitamin C used to be all the rage. Today, experts say it is best taken in your diet from foods such as citrus fruits and green vegetables. In one study, people with a high diet of vitamin C-rich foods had a much decreased risk of developing OA. Usual dose, if you need a supplement: 100–1,000mg per day.

VITAMIN D

Vitamin D is needed to help process calcium and build strong bones, and may help slow the progression of OA. In one study, OA was found to progress much faster in those with low levels of the vitamin. It can be made by our bodies when they're exposed to sunshine. Deficiencies are fairly common in many elderly people, especially those who live in northern climates. Usual dose: 400–800 IU per day.

VITAMIN E

This blood-thinning vitamin is promoted for heart health, but studies for arthritis are mixed. In some it eased OA and RA pain, but in others it did not. May increase bleeding risks. Usual dose: 400–600 IU per day.

VITAMIN E
The seeds of sunflowers are an excellent source of vitamin E, which is good for heart health. They may also help to relieve pain.

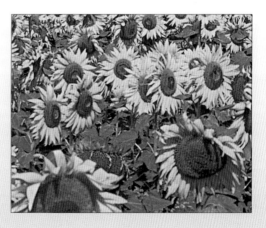

Exercising for health

If exercise came in a pill, it would be a miracle treatment. Study after study shows that it is essential for overall health and can make a major improvement in your arthritis symptoms. In fact, lack of exercise can add to pain and contribute to depression.

Doctors used to think that moving diseased joints would damage them more. Now we know it's essential to keep moving to build up the muscles that hold joints in place and to help pump nutrients into cartilage. Exercise also improves mood, eases pain and relieves depression.

But it can hurt to get moving when you have arthritis and some kinds of exercise can stress vulnerable joints. Ask your doctor or physiotherapist before doing any strenuous exercise or if your arthritis is severe or very painful. If you cannot walk by yourself, you can still get the benefits from exercise programmes designed to be done with a walker or from a chair or bed – even seated in the bath.

The fundamentals of fitness

Exercising for fitness means working to retain and improve your general health. Fitness and medical experts agree that an exercise programme should fulfil several basic objectives: it needs to increase or preserve flexibility, build strength and work the cardio–respiratory (heart and lungs) system. It should also include weight–bearing exercises, which help strengthen your bones and movements to help improve balance and coordination.

Flexibility

Flexibility in joints and muscles is like the suspension system in your car: it helps you travel better over bumps and rough terrain. Staying flexible helps your balance and your ability to adapt to different positions and postures. Flexibility exercises reduce stiffness and help keep joints mobile, which in turn relieves pain.

The normal amount joints can be moved in certain directions is called range-of-motion. Exercises that take your joints and muscles through a full range of movement

---

GETTING MOVING

Pain may be making you reluctant or nervous about starting to exercise. The following activities are a few recommended low-risk ways to get moving:

* Walking – start off with 10 minutes a day and build up to 40 minutes or so.
* Aquatics – swim or join an aquatic exercise group in a heated pool.
* Feldenkrais – learn to use your body more efficiently.
* Yoga – build flexibility, strength and inner peace with a meditative Eastern practice.
* Tai chi – build strength and improve your balance in body, mind and spirit with the slow controlled movements of this safest of exercises.

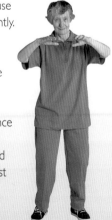

gradually increase both the extent and the ease of movement, so your joints, muscles and tendons operate with less pain and less likelihood of strain. Range–of–motion exercises usually include stretching, and are particularly useful first thing in the morning and when your joints are painful.

Strength

We need strong muscles to hold our joints in place and to keep them functioning properly. When your joints are damaged, as with many kinds of arthritis, it is important to keep muscles as strong as possible to support and protect those joints.

Lack of exercise quickly leads to weak muscles, which can result in joints that are out of alignment. Pain can cause "guarding" ways of moving that add even more stress. This extra stress and muscle weakness can, in turn, increase pain and may accelerate arthritis damage.

Several studies have shown that exercise can relieve the pain of OA of the knees. Improved muscle function may also delay or prevent the need for joint replacement. And if you need joint replacement, you need strong muscles more than ever, to support the new joints.

Many well–known athletes have OA as a result of sports injuries, yet they are able to perform at peak levels because their strong muscles protect their joints. Their OA may only bother them after retirement from active sports, when their training lapses and all the muscles protecting those joints become weaker.

EASING ACHES AND PAINS

The old standby hot-water bottle is good, as is the newer flexible hot pack that can be heated and reheated in a microwave. Reusable cold packs come in many shapes and sizes and can be kept in the freezer.

When using these products take care not to injure your skin and nerves. Always place a cloth between the hot or cold pack and your skin (some products come with a fabric covering). Only leave packs on for 20 minutes at a time. You might want to alternate heat and cold.

Hot tubs or Jacuzzis, with pulsing jets of warm water, can ease aches and may be worth the investment for your home. Hot wax in paraffin baths is another pain reliever especially good for hands. Special kits are available to prepare the wax, into which you dip hands. The wax stays on the area until it cools, keeping in the heat.

WARMING UP AND COOLING DOWN

Before exercising be sure to warm up – this will increase the blood supply to your muscles and joints, and get you ready to move. And after exercise don't stop abruptly – remember to cool down.

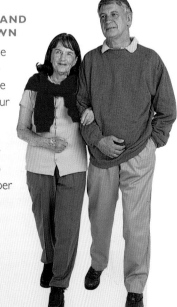

The way to strengthen your muscles is to use them regularly, gradually increasing the load. You don't have to start out with some heavy-duty exercise, either: just start to move, a little bit at a time.

Cardio-respiratory function

Improving your cardio-respiratory fitness helps to strengthen your heart and lungs and increases stamina, which is important for maintaining overall health.

The relevant exercises are commonly called aerobic, because they use large muscle groups in continuous movement to stimulate blood flow through your body. This has the effect of making your heart and lungs work harder and your muscles work more efficiently.

Aerobic exercises decrease risk of heart disease, high blood pressure and diabetes, and help to control weight, improve sleep and build up stamina.

But that does not mean you have to do joint-pounding, high-impact aerobics dance classes to get the benefits. Any exercise that makes you breathe more deeply and increases your pulse rate and circulation will do. That includes such joint-friendly workouts as walking, dancing, tai chi, swimming, water aerobics and riding a stationary bicycle.

Weight bearing

This does not mean you have to hoist a heavy weight or push a workout machine. It means you need to put some weight-type stress on your bones to keep them strong. Studies have shown that women with osteoporosis bone loss can slow or even stop bone loss by doing weight-bearing exercises. These could include routines with small hand weights of 5lb (2.3kg) or less or it could involve using the weight of your body in movement programmes, such as walking, dancing and tai chi.

Balance and coordination

Many doctors and therapists believe there is another objective for exercise: it should support correct body posture and use. It stands to reason that when your posture is correct, there will be less inappropriate wear of the joints and muscles. Balance will be better, and efficient body use can improve coordination and spatial awareness – knowing where your body is in relationship to other people and objects.

Your joints do not work as isolated units but rather as moving parts of a whole functioning body. When your posture is upright and aligned it takes less effort for you to move. Also, the lung space is larger (try to take a big breath and straighten your chest, you will notice there is more space in the chest).

Exercising safely

Anyone who has arthritis or a related musculoskeletal condition needs to take care with all movements – and especially exercise programmes aimed at improving fitness. Here are some guidelines to help you play it safe:

• Get a diagnosis so you are sure exactly what type of arthritis you have, and how it is affecting your joints and muscles. Don't just assume you have OA because of pain and stiffness.

• Before you start ask your doctor for an overall medical check-up, especially if you are very overweight, have been inactive for a long time, are a smoker or have high blood pressure, heart disease or another serious chronic condition.

• Ask a physiotherapist for an evaluation and advice for an exercise that suits you. Even people with the same conditions – for example OA of the knee – may have very different bodies and levels of physical condition. Find out what type of exercise, activity or sport a rehabilitation expert recommends for you.

• Start slowly. Some people with arthritis, who have been active all of their lives, find it very hard not to push too much.

Remember that this is not a competition. A quick-fix blitz is not appropriate. You are in this for long-term gains.

• Warm up before you exercise and cool down afterwards. No matter how gentle the exercise, take the time to prepare your body with some stretching, range-of-motion or other warming-up routine. Use similar measures at the end of the session to allow your body to gradually return to its normal state.

• Be "here now". Concentrate on the activity you are engaged in. Experts say that you will receive much more benefit from an

EXERCISE MACHINES
Always get expert advice about a routine that is safe for you before exercising on a machine.

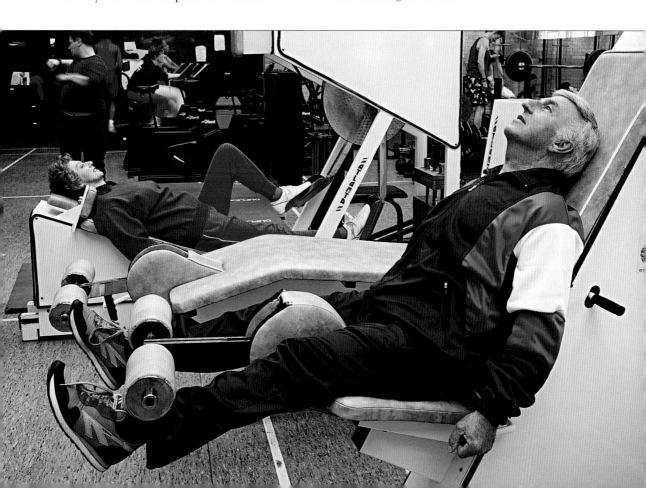

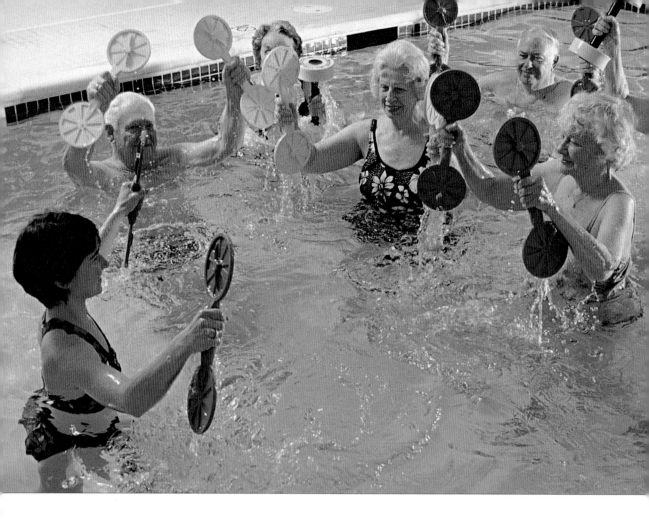

WATER AEROBICS

Water relieves the pull of gravity and may allow you to exercise with less pain and more enjoyment. Water aerobics can help improve stamina and muscle tone and reduce the risk of injuries.

exercise when you are bringing all of your attention to the movements. Listening to talk shows or the news, watching TV or using other distractions cuts into the mind–body benefits. It can also lead to injuries, since you are not paying proper attention to your movements.

* Stop any activity or exercise that causes you pain – in your joints, muscles or anywhere else in your body. Always do what is comfortable for you. If you experience chest pains, shortness of breath or dizziness, then you must call your doctor right away.

* Listen to your body. It is normal to have some discomfort after beginning an exercise, but if it lasts more than about two hours or you remain exhausted into the next day, you have probably done too much. (If this happens be sure to consult your doctor.) Alternatively, this may not be the right kind of exercise to you.

* Listen to your feelings. You should enjoy exercise. If you hate it, you simply won't do it regularly or with full attention. So experiment until you find something you really do enjoy.

Creating your personal exercise programme

Not all forms of exercise will interest you – and more important, not all of them will benefit you. Your own particular choice of exercise programme depends on various things, such as your current level of health and fitness, the limits of your physical ability, what you want to achieve and what activities you enjoy.

The severity of your arthritis, and any co–existing health problems you may have, will also determine what kind and how much movement you should be doing. You can create your own individual exercise programme, based on what appeals to you, what you can easily do and what you will do regularly.

Different activities appeal to different people. You may want to participate in the camaraderie of other people in a class or perhaps you prefer to work at your own pace in the gymnasium. Maybe an evening walk is a good time to catch up on family

MOTIVATION FOR MOTION

Getting started is often the easier part of an exercise routine. Keeping up the routine can be the hardest part. Even the most strong-willed person can find it difficult to exercise, day after day. Here are some tips to keep going:

- **Keep an exercise diary:** it helps to note each time you do your exercises and how you felt.
- **Make it a habit:** set the same time each day for your exercise, in the same place if possible, so that it becomes a routine.
- **Get support:** join a class, ask friends to join you, tell friends you are working out – do what you need to get others involved in helping you feel good about exercise.
- **Set goals and reward yourself:** this can be as simple as allowing yourself a treat after you work out, or a long-term goal to get into shape for a special holiday that requires lots of walking and energy, for example.
- **Change if you need to:** if you find out, after a trial of a few weeks, that an exercise isn't working for you – for example, the chlorine in the swimming pool irritates your eyes, or you hate the music in the aerobics class –

then don't do it. There is a whole world of different activities that can help you stay fit.
- **Cross-train:** this fancy term simply means adding variety to your workouts by doing different types of exercise that use different sets of muscles and mental skills. Otherwise, you will be using the same type of movements again and again and so may over-load a joint or muscle group.
- **Jazz it up:** music to move by – whether it's Mozart or Motown – can help carry you through exercise sessions at home. You could warm up first by walking on the spot (see *right*). There are special recordings made for every type of exercise, including tai chi and yoga.

news or a swim by yourself allows time out from the daily hassles. Choose activities that you can easily incorporate into your daily or weekly routine.

Enjoyment is important because an exercise programme will be a long-term commitment. It doesn't matter how good a programme is if you don't do it. Here is a review of some exercise options.

Home exercises

These daily workouts usually include flexibility and some strengthening exercises and are just right as a warm up for another part of your exercise programme, such as practising your tai chi or going for a walk. Physiotherapists often provide suggestions for a daily routine and can help you design a warm up for your particular needs.

Aerobic dance classes

These classes range from high–energy, high–impact workouts not suited for people with arthritis, to low–impact and even chair–based routines. There may be classes on offer at your local fitness, health or community centre. The classes may also be organized through senior citizen and adult education programmes as well as by your local arthritis organization.

EXERCISING TOGETHER
The enjoyment and camaraderie of doing a class with other people, especially outside in the fresh air, may make you more likely to exercise.

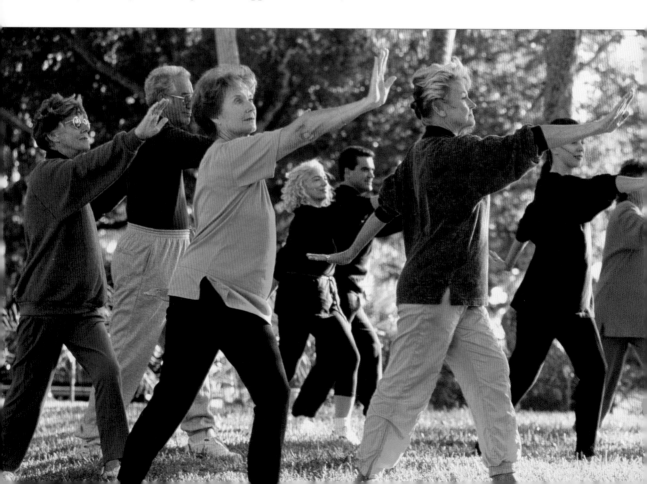

Some classes will concentrate mainly on gentle stretching and strengthening; others will include an aerobic component. All are enhanced by the group atmosphere and a cheerful and motivating teacher.

You may want to visit several aerobic dance classes to find one that suits you best and doesn't demand too much from you. In some countries you will find specially accredited senior fitness leaders or gentle exercise leaders.

Water exercise

Sometimes called aqua aerobics or aquacise, these exercise classes are held in warm-water swimming pools where you can work out without the drag of gravity. Some provide gentle general exercise, others aim to improve aerobic fitness. Your local arthritis organization may be able to direct you to a suitable class.

Movement re-education classes

The Feldenkrais method and the Alexander technique are two movement re-education programmes which have been designed to help people become more aware of their bodies and find the most efficient and pain-free ways of moving. They will require you to commit considerable time and effort but the benefits are worth it (*see page 71*).

Mind/body movement

The ancient practices of yoga and tai chi work body and mind and have a strong meditation component built into the carefully designed movement and breathing sequences. These are excellent for almost anyone, but be sure to choose an instructor or class designed for people with arthritis and other musculoskeletal conditions.

Yoga and tai chi are easy and fun to learn, and with only a few minutes of daily practice you can improve your arthritis and the quality of your life. The Tai Chi for Arthritis programme described in Chapters 5 and 6 was created specifically for people with musculoskeletal conditions.

Health clubs or gymnasiums

These fitness-oriented organizations offer a wide variety of exercise programmes and feature resistance equipment to tone up your muscles. Although these machines can help you build muscle strength, proceed with caution. Ask your doctor for advice before starting a fitness programme.

Don't depend on the instructors to help and advise you unless they have special training in working with people with musculoskeletal problems. They are usually trained only to work with healthy bodies, and so can give instructions that may be harmful. Avoid working with weights if your joints become easily inflamed.

General aerobic exercise

Aerobic exercise includes activities such as walking, swimming, cycling and dancing, or tennis, bowling and golf. All are easily accessible recreational pursuits that you can often enjoy with family and friends in pleasant surroundings.

Begin slowly, taking care not to go beyond your pain limits. Gradually build up aerobic fitness by increasing distance, speed or effort. Before you set off, warm up with some flexibility exercises.

Getting support

Living with arthritis can be a challenge. Sometimes it can be overwhelming. You can begin to meet some of the challenges by making your health your top priority. You can improve your well-being and take control of your arthritis – and not let your arthritis control you.

Try some of the suggestions listed here. You can also make the time to learn all about your particular type of arthritis and the many ways to improve your condition. Keep up with new developments in the medical world (*see Chapter Three*). Knowing about your arthritis and its treatments will make it easier for you to talk to your doctor and other health professionals about the progress of your symptoms and about the best treatments available.

Contact an arthritis organization about programmes for self-care and exercise (*see Resources, page 138*). Called "self-help" or "self-care", these programmes are designed to show people with chronic illness how to get the most out of life. They teach skills to make day-to-day tasks easier and strategies to help you to stay active. You learn how to cope better, both mentally and physically, with the changes in your life. They include tips on everything from dealing with emotional stress to finding assistive devices to help out in the kitchen (*see page 47*).

Think about joining a support group and consider counselling – both are ways of discussing your needs and concerns with people who understand. Give your diet an overhaul (*see pages 28–35*) and do what you can to take the stress out of your life. Consider trying out complementary therapies (*see pages 62–73*). And get moving: those joints were made for action.

FINDING A SUPPORT GROUP

Support groups and group therapy can make a great difference to the quality of your life.

Support groups will give you the reassurance that you are not alone. You will also get good advice on coping with arthritis from others in the group.

Your doctor may be able to direct you to a local support group. Arthritis organizations in many communities are good sources for finding a support group, as is your community centre or health clinic.

Support groups

Living with a chronic illness can become very lonely. No matter how much your family and friends sympathize, they don't really know what you are going through. Eventually, you may even find that people simply don't want to hear about your condition any more. You might find you're becoming isolated as you reduce the social events and activities you once enjoyed so consider joining a support group (*see left*).

Consider counselling

A quite normal effect of a chronic ailment is that people find they become depressed or that many emotional issues come to the

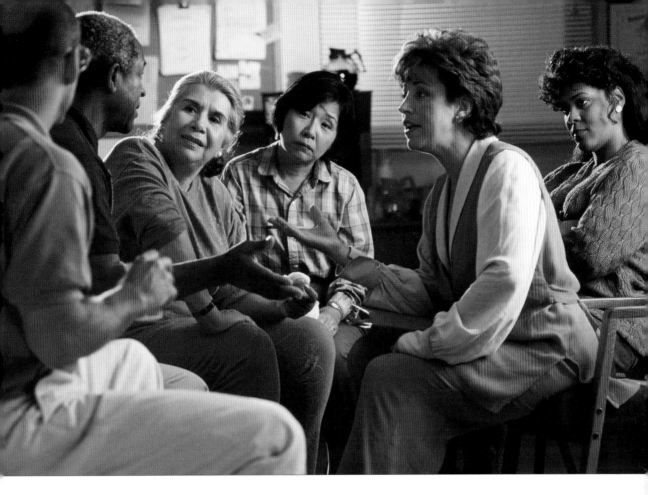

surface and are hard to cope with or understand. It's normal for someone who has developed a debilitating illness to feel a sense of loss. It's also normal to grieve for the many changes that a chronic illness can make in your life.

If you find that you are consistently feeling down and depressed for more than a month, and that you are having trouble coping with all of the changes in your life, you might want to seek counselling.

Talking things over with a mental health professional – someone who has special training to work with people who have chronic ailments – can help you cope better with these changes and the upheavals your emotions are going through.

THE BENEFITS OF A SUPPORT GROUP
Studies show that people with chronic illness who attend support groups tend to respond much better to treatment and feel better about themselves.

Stay involved

Let's face it: there are days when you don't want to see anyone, especially if you are in pain, or if your medication or arthritis symptoms have changed your appearance. But staying at home alone can become a habit – a habit that can increase your pain, depression and feelings of sadness.

Look for a support group (*see left*) where you can speak openly and honestly about how you feel. And do keep up with your friends and activities as much as you can. Many activities can be adapted to take into account that you may not be as mobile as you once were. Make a point to invite a friend for a meal: you can go to a restaurant so you don't have to cook. If you like gardening or exercising there's no need to stop. There are special tools and aids for gardening and many special exercise classes where you may meet new friends.

Ask for help when you really need it. Friends and family often want to help, but may avoid you because they don't know how to be of assistance. Their support can make it easier to cope, but you have to tell people that you need their help.

Avoid stress

Stress is such a problem in today's world that some even consider it an illness in its own right. It is known to contribute to heart disease and many other conditions, including arthritis flares.

Until perhaps a hundred years ago, stress played an important function. It prepared

CAUTION

Some helpful and assistive devices, such as the easy-open medicine lids and easy-grip car keys, may present a danger to small children and toddlers. They make potentially dangerous items accessible to little fingers which cannot open ordinary jars and doors.

This can be especially dangerous if you no longer have young children at home, and so may not be alert to potential problems. Be sure all your medicines, supplements, herbs and vitamins are safely stored out of the reach of children.

us to face up to physical dangers and compete physically. Today, we don't need to outrun wild animals or fight attacking enemies. But our primitive brain is still stuck with the "flight or fight" response, pushing our buttons in many odd and inappropriate situations.

Stress has little purpose today, but that doesn't keep us from feeling it. Many health clinics and hospitals now have stress reduction programmes that teach us how to recognize and let go of our tension and anxiety. These programmes usually combine daily exercise, meditation and relaxation training. They are well worth exploring.

SUPPORT FROM FAMILY AND FRIENDS
When coping with your arthritis becomes too much and stress takes over and overwhelms you, turn to your family, friends or someone you love, and be reminded how powerful a sympathetic ear can be.

USEFUL AND ASSISTIVE DEVICES

Movements and activities that once were so easy become a major struggle. Arthritis of the hands may make it impossible for you to cook or button a shirt. Knee or hip pain and stiffness can leave you trapped in an easy chair – or worse, on the toilet or in the bath. Arthritis in the shoulder, neck and elbow can make it painful to type, reach up or even talk on the phone. Here are some of the many products to help with the challenges of daily living.

DRESSING AIDS

- Zipper pulls, button hooks and other devices that will help you deal with small objects and openings.
- Brassieres with easy-to-fasten front fastenings. Velcro fastenings on clothes, shoes and other wardrobe items.

KITCHEN AIDS

- Rubber sheets for gripping lids better.
- Tong-type jar openers.
- Kitchen tools, such as peelers, with thicker, softer handles.

FOR MORE MOBILITY

- A walking stick can offer extra support to sore hips and knees – and be a fashion statement as well.
- Walkers, which now come with built-in seats in bright colours.

HOME IMPROVEMENTS

- Grab bars for bathrooms and raised toilet seats to make getting up and down easier.
- Lift chairs and lift seats that help push you up from sitting – including one for the toilet.
- Door handles, in place of knobs, that can be worked with pressure of the whole hand.
- Electric garage and other door openers.
- Door handle, switch and key enlargers to make these essential items easier to grasp.

NOTHING SPECIAL

Everyday products that are already arthritis-friendly.

- Flip-top caps. Many medications, cosmetics and cooking condiments come with large, flip-top caps that are much easier to open than screw caps.
- Carpenter's apron. This many-pocketed apron can save steps by giving you lots of pockets to carry items.
- Lightweight appliances. Look for smaller, lighter versions of electric tin openers, hand-held mixers and hair dryers.
- Easy-grip pens. Many shops now carry pens with wider, softer shafts that are easier to grip and use.
- Speaker telephone with voice-activated dialling or speed dialling.
- Telephone head sets to prevent neck and shoulder stress.
- Light switches activated by voice or sound.
- Book holders to avoid putting stress on your wrists.
- Special computer keyboards or voice-activated writing programmes.
- Long-handled "grabbers" that allow you to get items from high shelves or low places without bending or reaching.

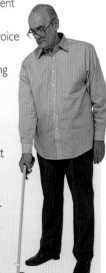

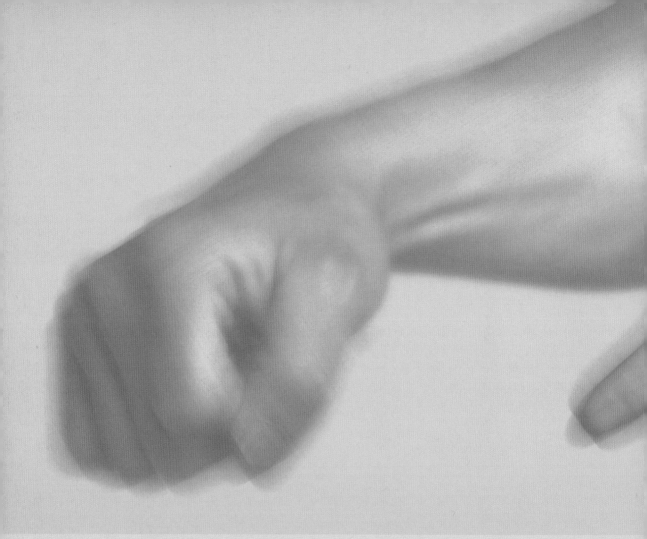

Treating
arthritis

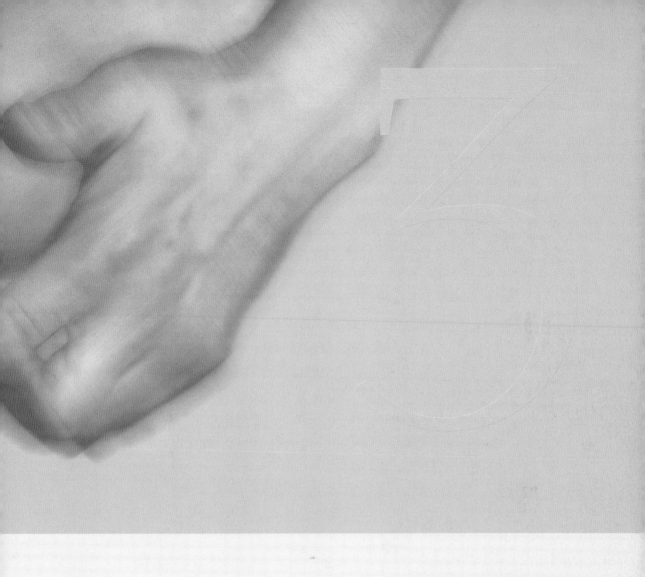

Researchers continue to investigate and discover new medications and therapies for treating arthritis. Doctors are also finding evidence that "alternative" therapies may complement conventional treatments for easing pain and other symptoms.

What Western medicine offers

Only a few decades ago, doctors and patients alike despaired at a diagnosis of arthritis. There were few effective treatments and no way to stop the progression of the most aggressive and crippling forms, such as rheumatoid arthritis. But researchers are increasingly developing new treatments to slow down or even stop severe joint damage, and are working on ways to repair or replace damaged cartilage and joints.

Today, there is still no cure for most kinds of arthritis. But advances in medicine have brought many new treatments. The most progress has been made in treating the inflammation of rheumatoid arthritis. Doctors may prescribe powerful immune-suppressant medicines, such as corticosteroids, to slow or halt inflammation. Most exciting of all is the creation of a whole new class of drugs called biologic response modifiers. These BRMs directly interfere with the production of inflammation by blocking the process that stimulates it.

There are also drugs available to prevent or replace the bone loss of osteoporosis, a problem for many with arthritis. The agonizing pain of gout can be treated and prevented with medications to increase output of uric acid and researchers are developing a new, hormone-based drug for lupus.

We don't know yet how to stop or replace the cartilage loss from osteoarthritis, the most common kind of arthritis. But drugs can help with pain, and researchers are looking at ways to grow replacement cartilage, or to stimulate your body to repair this valuable joint cushion. Total joint replacement has been very successful: when joints can no longer function, doctors can replace them with artificial joints.

Doctors also advise people with any kind of arthritis to maintain a healthy weight to avoid putting extra stress on muscles and joints; to exercise regularly; to eat a balanced, low-fat diet; and to avoid physical and mental stress, which can cause flares and worsen symptoms. Self-help programmes sponsored by arthritis organizations, including Arthritis Care, offer group support and techniques that make it easier to live with arthritis.

There is growing acceptance of many ancient and so–called "alternative" therapies. These are known as complementary therapies when they are used to support conventional Western treatments. Moreover, there is increasing evidence for the role that mind and spirit can play in both illness and health.

Using a combination of conventional medications, complementary therapies, self–help guidance and exercise routines, you can take control of your arthritis and not let your arthritis control you.

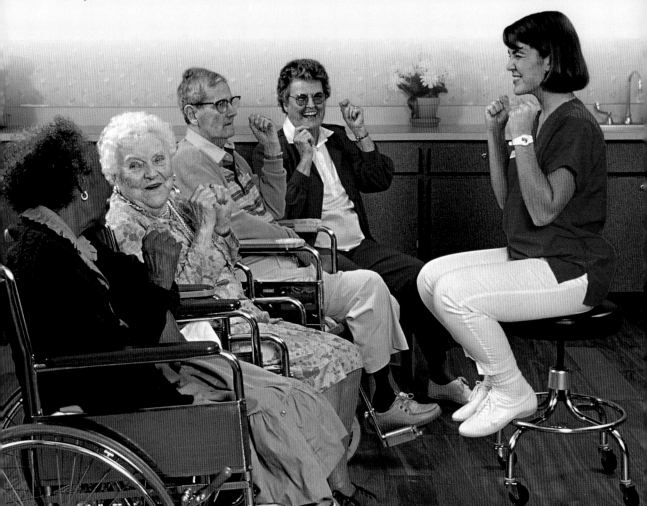

Easing pain and inflammation

Pain is often the worst symptom for people with arthritis, a constant companion that keeps you from sleeping, exercising, even eating. Inflammation often, but not always, comes with pain and, if left unchecked, can cause permanent joint damage.

When your joints are aching, the first thing you are likely to reach for is such over-the-counter pain or inflammation medications as aspirin or paracetamol. You might also try ibuprofen, the prescription drugs ketoprofen or naproxen sodium, or one of the many ointments advertised to ease joint pain (*see right*).

And no wonder: these workhorse drugs remain the mainstay for many with arthritis. For those whose symptoms are minor to moderate, these basic medicines may be enough. For those people with severe arthritis, these medicines may be taken in their stronger prescription format, or along with powerful disease-modifying drugs.

For pain only: analgesic drugs

Turn to the following treatments when pain relief is your main goal:

Paracetamol

This popular drug is available under many brand names. It is aspirin-free and so can be taken by those people who are allergic to aspirin and by young children who may develop reactions to aspirin products. Take as directed on the bottle or by your doctor.

Caution: drinking alcohol at the same time as taking paracetamol has been known to cause liver damage.

Narcotic drugs

When your pain is severe, or after surgery or other procedures, your doctor may prescribe powerful narcotic pain relievers. Among the most common used for arthritis pain are oxycodone, hydrocodone with paracetamol, codeine with paracetamol or tramadol.

Caution: these must be taken as directed as they can be habit-forming. Do not drink alcohol when taking them as it can dangerously increase their effects.

Pain-easing ointments

It feels natural to want to rub out that ache, and there are ointments and creams that can help interrupt pain, albeit for a short time. Marketed under many names and formulas, there are three main types of pain-relieving ointment.

• Ointments containing capsaicin, which is the compound that gives chilli peppers their bite. Capsaicin interferes with a chemical that conducts pain messages.

• "Counter-irritant" ointments, which contain one or more substances, such as menthol, camphor or the oils of wintergreen or eucalyptus. These substitute a feeling of heat or cool for pain.

• Salicylate ointments, which contain aspirin-like ingredients that ease pain and inflammation.

Caution: while generally safe, any of these ointments might irritate the skin and should never be used around the eyes or other sensitive areas. Be sure to wash your hands thoroughly after applying.

To ease pain and inflammation

When your joints are swollen, hot or inflamed, these drugs may help:

Non-steroidal anti-inflammatory drugs (NSAIDs)

NSAIDs help to reduce inflammation and control pain. They are among the most widely used medicines for treating arthritis. Ibuprofen is an NSAID available over the counter; naproxen sodium, ketoprofen and the stronger NSAIDs indomethacin and diclofenac are prescribed by doctors. Here are some other types of NSAID:

◆ Aspirin belongs to a subcategory called salicylates and has the added advantage of offering protection against some kinds of heart disease.

◆ An NSAID ointment to be applied just to the sore joint is available in some countries: it uses a transdermal agent to carry diclofenac through the skin.

◆ COX2 inhibitors, such as celecoxib and rofecoxib, are a new kind of NSAID. They block the COX2 enzymes that produce the inflammation–causing prostaglandins but don't affect the biochemical process that protect the stomach and intestines.

They are much more expensive than the usual NSAIDs but are important for people at risk from internal bleeding or who are taking blood–thinning drugs. However, as with NSAIDs, the COX2 inhibitors may contribute to kidney problems. They do not offer the heart protection of a daily aspirin, and there is some concern they may contribute to clotting in some people.

NSAIDS: USE WITH CAUTION

The non-steroidal anti-inflammatory drugs (NSAIDs) can be truly wonder drugs, easing pain for millions of people and available almost everywhere. But not even aspirin – the first NSAID – is completely safe. Thousands of people die every year from NSAID complications, such as gastrointestinal bleeding, ulcer disease and kidney damage.

The older we are, the more vulnerable we become to the side effects of aspirin and NSAIDs. We've been taking these drugs longer and we may also be taking blood-thinning and other drugs that multiply the side effects. People who take supplements or herbs that are blood-thinners, such as garlic, ginkgo and ginger, are also at added risk, as are people who drink alcohol.

Take all medications with caution and follow the instructions on the pack of those you can buy without a prescription.

BLOOD-THINNING SUBSTANCES

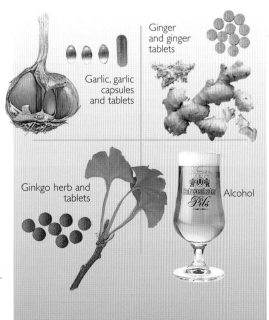

Ginger and ginger tablets

Garlic, garlic capsules and tablets

Ginkgo herb and tablets

Alcohol

Attacking inflammation at the source

The symptoms of arthritis can be eased with pain relievers and anti–inflammatory agents. But the destructive process of the auto–immune and inflammatory types of arthritis often continue, doing permanent damage to joints and sometimes to internal organs. This can lead to disability and even death in severe cases. Powerful drugs may slow or stop that process by attacking inflammation at its source. These drugs can also have strong side effects and so are used for the more severe types of arthritis.

Corticosteroids

These are powerful prescription anti–inflammatory drugs for rheumatoid arthritis, lupus and other types of arthritis. Among the corticosteroids used for arthritis are cortisone, prednisolone, methylprednisolone and hydrocortisone.

Corticosteroids were first derived from cortisol, a hormone produced naturally by our adrenal glands. They were hailed as "miracle drugs" when first developed since cortisone suppresses inflammatory disease activity in, and reduces the body's auto–immune response to, various conditions.

However, it was soon discovered that the drugs can have serious side effects with long–term use. Among the most serious are cataracts, osteoporosis (*see box, page 55*) and a susceptibility to infection. Other side effects include weight gain, acne, thinning of skin tissue, facial hair growth and mental and mood changes. Corticosteroids may also mask signs of infection and their use has to be gradually tapered off.

While still a major weapon against auto–immune disease, corticosteroids are used more cautiously today. Doctors prescribe the lowest dose possible to control inflammation. But stronger doses can be important weapons against very severe cases of arthritis that can be destructive and even fatal, and to prevent organ damage during flares.

To improve mobility, cortisone injections are sometimes given directly into a very inflamed area, such as a rheumatoid or osteoarthritic joint, often giving significant relief for several months.

Disease–modifying anti–rheumatic drugs (DMARDs)

A number of very powerful arthritis drugs, known collectively DMARDs, don't just treat symptoms but can actually modify the inflammation process. They may slow the progression of rheumatoid arthritis, psoriatic arthritis, ankylosing spondylitis and certain other rheumatic diseases, sometimes even bringing about a remission.

Among the oldest DMARDs are solutions containing gold, which are taken orally or given in injections. Other DMARDs, which have now been found to be effective for inflammatory kinds of arthritis, were originally developed for other conditions: methotrexate was developed to treat cancer; cyclosporine to prevent the rejection of organ transplants; hydroxychloroquine as a treatment for malaria. Recently, new drugs such as leflunomide were developed specifically to combat RA.

In the past, doctors used to wait until all other treatments failed before starting a course of these powerful drugs. Now DMARDs are prescribed aggressively in the early stages of severe arthritis, either to slow or prevent permanent joint damage.

Often DMARDs are used in combination treatments. They may take a month or more to show an effect. They are not all equally effective for everyone and can have serious side effects. Ask your doctor about vitamins or supplements that might offset some of the effects (*see Folic acid, page 35*).

Biologic response modifiers

Biologic response modifiers (BRMs, or biologic agents) are a new class of drug that block the production of substances that can cause inflammation. Some interfere with the action of tumour necrosis factor (TNF), a protein believed to play a big role in causing inflammation and joint damage.

Among these new drugs that block the action of TNF are infliximab and etanercept. Infliximab has also been approved for Crohn's disease and is used for some cases of psoriatic arthritis. Etanercept has been approved for use in adults and young children. BRMs are being developed that block the action of other inflammatory agents, such as interleukin–1 (IL–1).

BRMs reduce bone and cartilage damage in RA. Used alone or combined with other drugs, they are very effective for some people. However, they are expensive and may leave people vulnerable to infections. Their long–term side effects are unknown.

OSTEOPOROSIS: BONES AT RISK

Osteoporosis is a gradual loss of bone density that leaves bones so brittle and fragile they are easily fractured. These fractures are a major cause of disability and death, especially among the elderly. Older women are particularly vulnerable.

Bone loss is linked to both calcium deficiency and heredity: at special risk are women whose ethnic background is Northern European and who are post-menopausal, small-boned and slender. People with arthritis may also be at special risk. Osteoporosis can be a side effect of corticosteroids.

Several treatments can stop or slow bone weakness: calcium supplements, oestrogen replacement, vitamin D supplements and drugs, such as the bisphosphonates alendronate and risedronate, and parathyroid hormone injections. One of the best ways to prevent and treat osteoporosis is weight-bearing exercise, which can also help the symptoms of your arthritis.

This electron micrograph shows the loss of bone density in the spongy bone tissue of a vertebra affected by osteoporosis.

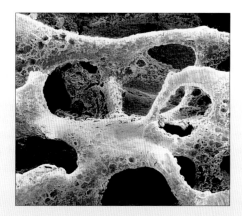

Prosorba therapy

This therapy filters the blood to remove the rheumatoid factor antibodies that are known to contribute to inflammation. Prosorba therapy may be used for people with RA who have not responded to other treatments. It is named after the filtering medium, a small cylinder that your blood passes through. In the process, which takes two to three hours, blood is taken from one arm, passed through the filtering machine, and then returned to your body through your other arm.

The treatment is carried out once a week for 12 weeks, usually at an outpatient centre. Some people experience an RA flare right after the treatment. But it can make RA inactive for a year or more.

Antibiotics therapy

It is known that infection, including Lyme disease, can cause arthritis and joint damage. Some rheumatologists believe that bacterial infections may cause some of the inflammatory kinds of arthritis, such as RA, scleroderma, ankylosing spondylitis and lupus, and even contribute to osteoarthritis. They prescribe low doses of antibiotics, particularly from the tetracycline family, such as minocycline, doxycycline and tetracycline. Antibiotics therapy is still being studied.

Fighting depression and pain

People with arthritis and chronic pain often become depressed or have trouble sleeping. This, in turn, contributes to more pain and further depression. Medications for the depression and specialists at chronic pain centres may help.

Antidepressants to the rescue

Illness can make us feel "blue". When the depression won't go away, an increasing number of medications can make a difference. Among the oldest are the tri-cyclic antidepressants, such as amitriptyline hydrochloride and nortriptyline. Newer medications, called selective serotonin reuptake inhibitors (SSRIs), increase the levels of your body's natural antidepressant, serotonin. Prozac (fluoxetine) is probably the best known. Antidepressants may also ease pain and help with sleep problems. Ask your doctor if you are depressed. She or he may prescribe one or more of these medications, along with exercise and perhaps some counselling.

People with fibromyalgia (*see page 21*) may be given low doses of antidepressants to help control pain and improve their sleep. Muscle relaxants, such as cyclobenzaprine or trazodone, may also help.

TENS treatments

TENS, which stands for transcutaneous electrical nerve stimulation, uses a small machine to relieve pain through mild electrical pulses. It is thought the electrical charges stimulate nerves and thus block pain impulses. Another theory is that TENS pulses stimulate the release of endorphins, the body's own feel-good hormones.

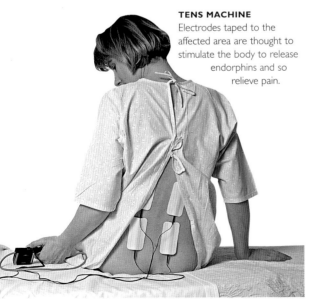

TENS MACHINE
Electrodes taped to the affected area are thought to stimulate the body to release endorphins and so relieve pain.

The TENS device comes with electrodes that are attached to the skin by tape over painful areas, and connected by wires to the TENS machine. The treatment may tingle but should not cause pain. The devices are available from some physio-therapists and doctors, and larger chemists.

When the pain becomes constant

Too often, we feel we have to just "tough it out" with pain. But experts look differently at the problem these days.

Acute pain – the kind we get from a cut, a burn or infection – is an alarm warning us to stop the painful activity and get treatment. But chronic pain – the kind that grinds on day after day such as that from arthritis – has no immediate purpose. And it can be debilitating.

Together, you and your doctor may be able to manage your chronic pain with a combination of medicines, exercise and counselling. When these fail to work, a referral to a chronic pain centre may be of some help.

Chronic pain centres

These centres usually take a team approach to helping people relieve pain that has become constant. Depending on your condition you may see one or more of the following: a neurologist, who specializes in the causes of pain; an anaesthetist, who specializes in pain medications; a physiotherapist and/or an occupational therapist; and a mental health practitioner such as a counsellor. Some pain clinics may also offer you massage, acupuncture and deep relaxation.

Improving mobility

Arthritis really hits home when it prevents us from moving with ease. Suddenly, the simplest chores, such as buttoning a shirt or walking downstairs, become painful or even impossible. Loss of mobility can threaten the ability to earn a living, to participate in activities and even our very independence. While medications can help a great deal, physiotherapy and, in severe cases, surgery can help to restore movement.

Seeing a movement specialist

When movement is an issue, therapists who specialize in body mechanics, such as a physiotherapist or occupational therapist, can be a great help, especially with everyday activities. A physiotherapist is trained in rehabilitating and conditioning bodies affected by injuries and disease. An occupational therapist can help you adapt to do everyday activities at home or work, such as dressing, cooking, housework and driving a car. Both can help you remain independent and even continue hobbies and recreational activities

These therapists can design an exercise programme specifically for you and your arthritis. They will analyze the way you move, note any biomechanical problems you may have that contribute to joint stress and give you a personalized exercise routine. They may also give ultrasound, a high–energy sound–wave treatment that can ease pain in joints and muscles.

If needed, they can fit you with a brace, splints or other supportive devices: even walking sticks should be "fitted" by a professional. A physiotherapist can help you reduce the risk of further injuring your joints, strengthen your muscles and help you cope with pain and disabilities.

Viscosupplementation

This therapy involves injecting fluids that mimic the body's own lubricants into the knee joint. They are primarily given to relieve the stiffness and pain from OA. Treatments consist of a series of injections over a period of a three to five weeks, and may give relief for six months to a year. So far, the injections are only given in the knee but are being studied for use in other joints.

These injections have been used in advanced cases of knee OA when other therapies don't help with pain, or to delay the need for joint surgery. Some research is showing that injections given early in the development of OA may help to slow the process of cartilage damage. However, other research shows the treatment is no better than a placebo. These injections don't work for everyone and, because they're made from rooster combs, need to be used with care by people with egg or feather allergies.

Repairing and replacing joints

Surgery can help relieve pain and restore mobility to joints damaged by arthritis. The options range from minor procedures to total joint replacement. Artificial joints are available for everything from your little finger joint to your hip. No surgery should be undertaken without careful consideration of the rehabilitation time and possible risks.

Arthroscopy

In this minimally invasive procedure, the surgeon inserts a small tube-like instrument into the joint to view the cartilage and joint surfaces in order to make a diagnosis. The surgeon may also use other small instruments to repair joint damage and to remove damaged tissue and debris from the joint. Arthroscopy is particularly successful for restoring mobility to joints that have been injured and may help in the early stages of OA. Recovery from the procedures is usually very quick.

Artificial cartilage

Researchers are working now with plastic and metal devices that can replace damaged and worn-away cartilage in knees where the joints are bone-to-bone.

One type of replacement is a smooth metal "spacer" that can be inserted inside the knee joints to allow them to pivot easily. Another implants a polyurethane product (called an elastomer) that acts more like cartilage and is custom fit for each patient.

These replacement procedures are not yet widely available, and not everyone is a candidate. Nor are they a subsitute for joint replacement, but are being considered as ways of delaying the need for total joint

ARTIFICIAL HIP
Replacing the hip joint has become an increasingly common operation with a good success rate. A high proportion of replacement hips still function well after many years.

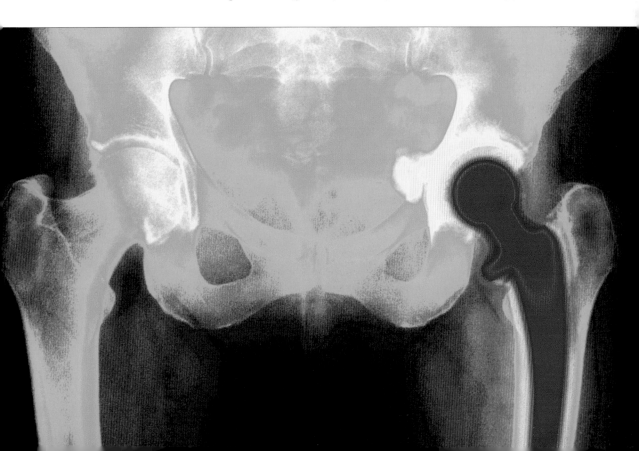

replacement in younger people, or for the elderly who might not want to undergo the long rehabilitation process of a total knee joint replacement.

Joint reconstruction

This surgical procedure may involve some of the other options discussed on these pages, together with the repair of tendons and ligaments to help improve the function of a joint. It is most commonly used in the joints of the hands and feet.

Vertebroplasty

This new procedure could help people whose vertebrae have collapsed or have been damaged by osteoporosis or fractures. The technique may also be used on hips or other bones to treat and prevent fractures.

A surgeon will make a small incision in the skin and then use a needle to inject a bone substitution material into the broken or weakened bones of the joint. Once this biodegradable material has hardened, it strengthens the bones.

TOMORROW'S TREATMENTS

New treatments, such as stem cell therapy and cartilage transplants, are being developed for many kinds of arthritis. Procedures for severe RA not generally available yet include bone marrow transplantation, in which your own bone marrow is removed, treated and returned.

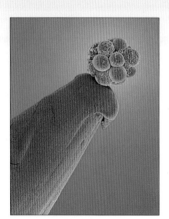

STEM CELL THERAPY

This therapy may eventually help diseased joints repair themselves. Researchers are working to direct stem cells – the immature cells in the body that haven't yet been dedicated to become part of a specific tissue – to develop into a particular type of cell. For example, they could become chondrocytes, the cells that generate cartilage. These cells could then grow into cartilage in the laboratory, which could be transplanted into damaged cartilage to spur new growth.

STEM CELLS

This electron micrograph shows a cluster of 10 almost identical, rounded stem cells of a human embryo on the tip of a pin. Each cell contains a central nucleus with the genetic instructions to become an adult human being.

CARTILAGE TRANSPLANTS

Cartilage can be transplanted from a part of your joint into the area damaged by arthritis. Researchers are also able to remove some of your cartilage and use it to grow more cartilage cells in a test-tube. The new cartilage is then put back into your injured joint. This technique is being used in some places to repair damaged cartilage in knee joints. However, only very tiny amounts of cartilage can be replaced in this way, and it is a very expensive procedure. It is generally regarded as effective for young people who have a cartilage injury and not yet for those who have lost cartilage through OA.

Total joint replacement

This procedure can be very successful in both relieving pain and restoring mobility to joints that have become diseased or damaged beyond repair. There are more joint replacement surgeries performed on the knee (*see box, right*) and hip than on any other joints. Most total joint replacements are for people with OA.

Operations to remove a damaged joint and replace it with an artificial implant made from hard–wearing plastic, metal or ceramics are very successful. Your doctor may suggest replacing all or part of a joint with an artificial joint if the damage from your arthritis gets to the point where it seriously interferes with your ability to move easily, causes pain so severe it wakes you at night, or deforms your joints.

Other surgical options

Osteotomy, resection and joint fusion are rarely used today for arthritis but they may be an option in some cases.

In osteotomy and resection, parts of the bone in a joint are cut away, or cut and then realigned. The procedures are used to correct bony deformities and so relieve stress on joints. They can help to relieve pain by redistributing weight and allowing easier movement of the joint. They may help slow the progress of OA caused by wear from bones that are out of line.

Joint fusion fixes the bones of a joint together and therefore prevents any further movement. It is a last resort procedure when all else fails and is usually used to reduce pain and improve the stability of a joint such as a wrist or ankle.

TOTAL KNEE JOINT REPLACEMENT

There are more than 150 different designs of joints for knee replacements.

In this operation, the opposing parts of the joint are replaced with a mechanical joint made of special metals, high-grade plastics and sometimes ceramic materials.

Surgeons used to prefer to replace joints on people who were approaching old age, as the joints had a useful life of about ten years or so. Today's knee joints have a 95 per cent chance of lasting 15 to 20 years, so they are an option for younger people as well.

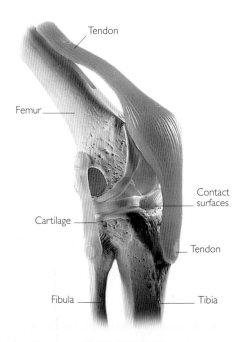

Tendon

Femur

Cartilage

Fibula

Contact surfaces

Tendon

Tibia

ARTIFICIAL KNEE JOINT
This shows an artificial total knee joint replacement. It is made of plastic and consists of new contact surfaces, an artificial cartilage between the faces and artificial tendons to limit flexion of the joint and to prevent sideways movement.

Beyond the medicine chest

There is no doubt that Western medicine excels at treating acute ailments such as infections, injuries and life-threatening conditions. But when it comes to ailments that have no cure, you may want to look beyond the medicine chest. Many treatments we consider alternatives, such as acupuncture and meditation, have been in use for thousands of years to treat arthritis. Some have few or no side effects and have helped many live better with long-term ailments.

Other so-called "alternative" therapies are finding their way into mainstream medicine. Physiotherapists recommend or use yoga, tai chi and movement re-education programmes to help people with arthritis, and massage is included in some rheumatology clinics. Herbs and homeopathy are used by millions of people. Therapeutic touch is accepted and used by more than 30,000 nurses in the United States alone.

As scientists begin to study these therapies, they are finding evidence that they can help ease pain, inflammation and other symptoms associated with arthritis, such as depression and insomnia. In fact, so many are entering Western medicine that they are called "complementary" – they are used alongside, but not in place of, conventional medicine.

Proceed with caution

Some alternative remedies and therapies are being accepted by doctors, but there are also many useless or even harmful ones – and unscrupulous people who promise to take away your pain but take only your money. Beware especially of the supplements advertised as "cures" in the media.

If you have an ailment or problem, see a doctor first for an examination and diagnosis. It's important to know exactly what you are treating. Always tell your doctor everything you are using or doing: your doctor needs to be informed about your total health situation and treatments.

Always check for side effects and interactions with other remedies – some treatments might harm you or interfere with your prescription drugs. Ask your doctor for a referral to a complementary therapist or find a therapist who is willing to keep your doctor informed. Before you begin a therapy, check the reputation and credentials of the therapist. Buy supplements or other remedies only from a reputable business.

Be very careful when combining several herbs and supplements: you don't know what the overall effect might be. Try the remedies or treatments one at a time, so you can tell what effect each has. Keep a diary of the treatments you try, so you can monitor the effects over time.

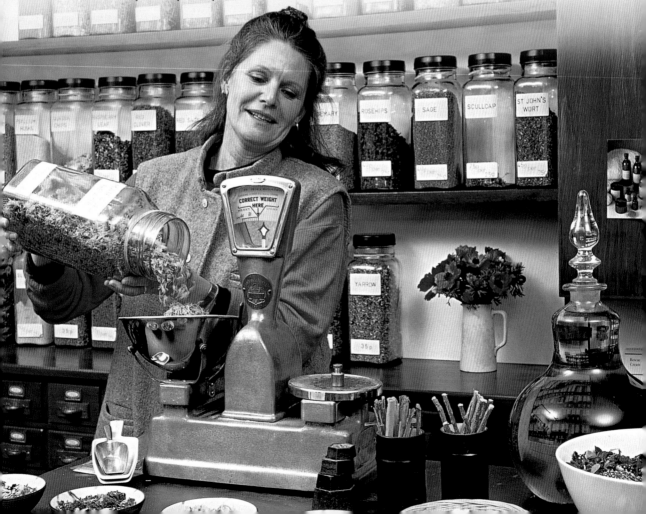

Mind–body medicine

We know that pain can affect the way we feel and that the way we feel emotionally can affect our level of pain. But people with long-term ailments can forget how the "mind–body connection" can be used to make us feel better physically and mentally. Indeed, many mind–body practices, such as meditation and biofeedback, are now so accepted by mainstream medicine that they are offered at hospitals and clinics.

Meditation

Meditation is an ancient practice that develops calmness and insight. While there are many different kinds, all help you quiet your mind to allow internal thoughts and external stimuli to flow by, without getting caught up in them. Regular practice of this technique has been shown to quieten your body as well. Studies show it can help relieve chronic pain, depression and stress, and ease fibromyalgia symptoms.

Some types of meditation focus on the silent repetition of a word, a sound or the feel of your own breathing. You may also meditate on a visual focus, such as a symbol, an image or a candle flame.

"Mindfulness meditation" – also known as *Vipassana* meditation – is said to cultivate a non-judgmental awareness of the present moment and is taught in many stress-reduction programmes.

Praying, in which a holy phrase or prayer is repeated, may be one of the oldest forms of meditation. But you don't have to believe in a religious or spiritual aspect of meditation to reap its benefits. Researchers have shown that focusing on a word or phrase – even the word "one" – can evoke a relaxed and peaceful mind and body.

Many organizations teach meditation and you can also learn to meditate from various non-religious books and a wide selection of audio tapes.

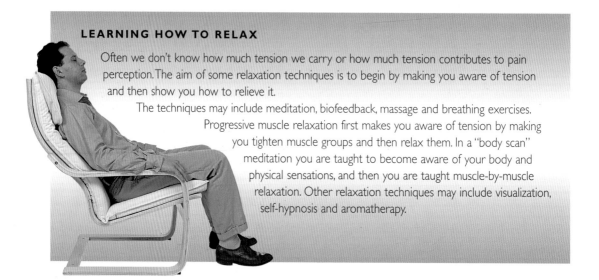

LEARNING HOW TO RELAX

Often we don't know how much tension we carry or how much tension contributes to pain perception. The aim of some relaxation techniques is to begin by making you aware of tension and then show you how to relieve it.

The techniques may include meditation, biofeedback, massage and breathing exercises. Progressive muscle relaxation first makes you aware of tension by making you tighten muscle groups and then relax them. In a "body scan" meditation you are taught to become aware of your body and physical sensations, and then you are taught muscle-by-muscle relaxation. Other relaxation techniques may include visualization, self-hypnosis and aromatherapy.

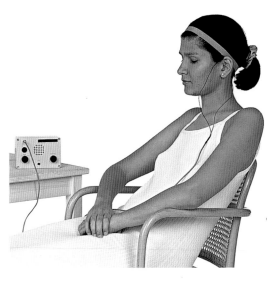

BIOFEEDBACK
Studies have shown that when you have learned a biofeed-back technique it can help ease stress and pain from several conditions, including RA.

Biofeedback

This technique uses electronic monitors to help you learn how your mind affects your body and how to change specific body functions. You are hooked up painlessly to instruments that measure pulse, heartbeat, body temperature or other processes.

A therapist helps you learn mind–body or relaxation techniques that can affect these processes. As you practise these, the electronic instruments "feedback" the effects on your body with light, sound or other signals. When you learn what techniques work for you, you can practise them without instruments.

Visualization and guided imagery

These techniques use the power of your imagination to take you to places or times where you are peaceful, pain-free and healthy. They help to relieve pain, promote relaxation and change behaviour patterns. You've probably used them already when a smell, sound or sight reminds you of a place or time where you felt happy, safe or loved.

To experiment with consciously using visualization, find a quiet place to sit or lie down. Now bring up a physical sensation and place that is soothing to you. If you enjoy the beach, evoke the smell of salt water, the sound of waves lapping on the shore and the sun's warmth on your skin.

In guided imagery, an audio or video tape leads you through a peaceful, pain-free experience. Many useful tape and books are available; or make your own tape with your own meaningful images and sensations.

Hypnotherapy

To many people, hypnosis conjures up stage shows where magicians make people from the audience perform silly actions against their will.

But hypnosis is really a very old type of mind-body therapy, a concentration technique that focuses your mind on a specific action or thought, allowing you to enter into a state of relaxed attention.

Psychotherapists use it to help people change behaviour or learn to relax, and it can help ease pain and stress. Studies show that people with fibromyalgia have less pain and fatigue and that people with arthritis have less pain, anxiety and depression.

Hypnotherapy is like guided imagery: you're led through deeper relaxation or into images of yourself as healthy and pain-free.

Touch & energy therapies

Touch can be powerful medicine, calming and soothing both physical and emotional "dis-ease". Massage has a long history of easing pain. Many kinds of touch therapy also involve the transmission of energy or the balancing of energy fields. In fact, some would say that healing energy passes between therapist and patient in almost all kinds of touch therapy. For that reason, the choice of a therapist can be of utmost importance in these very personal and intimate treatments.

Massage

This might well be the most basic of all therapies: massage has been used for thousands of years to ease pain and relieve muscle tension. We were all patted and soothed as babies, and most of us will instinctively rub an area that is hurting. A good massage can ease pain, relieve tight muscles and nerves, and promote welcome relaxation.

An increasing number of studies support the claims for the many benefits of massage. Perhaps most important for people with arthritis is evidence that massage can relieve pain and help restore mobility.

There are many styles and types of massage. Some, such as Swedish massage, involve stroking and kneading muscles. Others, such as shiatsu, apply deep pressure to different parts of the body and so effect healing. The type of massage is not as important as finding a massage therapist who is qualified to work with your kind of arthritis and who can ease your pain and muscle tension without injuring your joints.

Ask for a referral from your doctor or physiotherapist. Regardless of the massage therapist's credentials, only allow yourself to be massaged if it is comfortable and comforting; sometimes the pressure can aggravate your pain. Do not have a massage during a flare: hot, swollen joints should not be massaged.

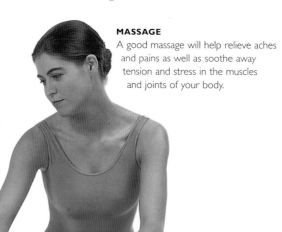

MASSAGE
A good massage will help relieve aches and pains as well as soothe away tension and stress in the muscles and joints of your body.

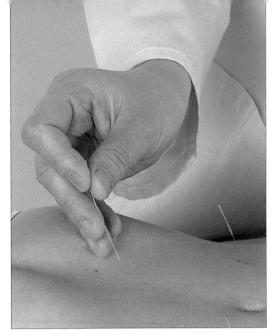

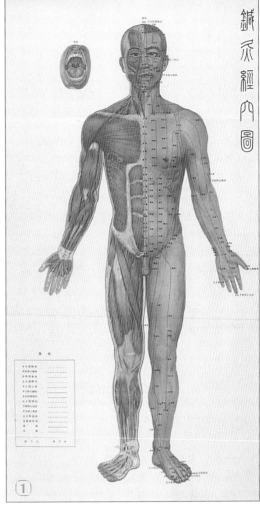

ACUPUNCTURE
Acupuncture treatments involve needles that enhance or balance the flow of *qi* through the dozen or so meridians of the body (*right*).

You can experiment with self–massage of aching joints and muscles. Use different pressures with your palm or fingers to find what soothes you. Better still, a friend or family member could learn some simple massage techniques.

Acupuncture and acupressure

Acupuncture originated in China thousands of years ago, and is based on balancing a person's vital life energy, called *qi* (*see The power of* qi, *pages 78–81*).

According to Traditional Chinese Medicine, *qi* flows through the body along invisible channels, called meridians. When the flow of *qi* is blocked or out of balance, illness or pain results. Practitioners of acupuncture and acupressure will stimulate specific points along the body's meridians to correct the flow of *qi* and so restore equilibrium and optimize health.

In acupuncture, hair–fine needles are inserted into the skin at specific acupoints which the practitioner chooses for your unique physical and mental situation. Only a few needles may be used or, in some cases, more than a dozen.

The points can also be stimulated with heat and herbs (called moxibustion), mild electrical current (electroacupuncture) and magnets. Acupressure is acupuncture without the needles: a practitioner uses fingers, hands, elbows and feet to apply pressure to selected acupoints.

Western science hasn't identified *qi* or any energy meridians, and researchers still don't know how acupuncture really works. However, research shows that acupuncture can stimulate several physical responses, including the release of endorphins, the body's feel-good hormones.

Several studies have revealed that acupuncture can ease pain, including OA pain as well as fibromyalgia symptoms and depression. To date there are few studies on acupressure available in English, but the therapy has been shown to relieve nausea and help with headaches.

Caution: both are generally regarded as safe when performed by a trained therapist. Check the credentials and training of the therapist before undergoing acupuncture, and be sure that only sterile needles are used to prevent any possibility of infection.

Foot reflexology

This therapy is sometimes referred to as foot massage, but it is more than that. Foot reflexologists believe the foot is a "mirror" of the body as a whole – different areas of the foot represent different organs and parts of the body.

Using the thumb or index finger, the reflexologist focuses on putting pressure on specific reflex points in the foot to stimulate healing in corresponding parts or functions of the body.

There are many health claims, but little scientifically accepted research. However, it is known that the feet have many nerve endings that can be stimulated or soothed by massage. Foot reflexology may contribute to relaxation and pain relief.

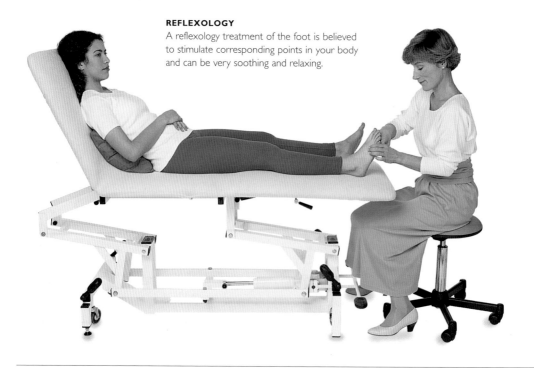

REFLEXOLOGY
A reflexology treatment of the foot is believed to stimulate corresponding points in your body and can be very soothing and relaxing.

Therapeutic touch

Developed in the 1960s in the United States by a professor of nursing, therapeutic touch has become widely used in hospitals and clinics across America.

The therapy is based on the unproven theory that we all possess unique fields of energy that interact with the environment and with one another. Illness can be caused by disturbances or imbalances in a person's energy field.

In therapeutic touch, the therapist does not actually touch you at all: the therapist first attunes to your energy field, and then moves his or her hands a few inches above your body, feeling for and balancing blockages in your energy field. Sweeping motions with the hands may be used to direct the patient's energy flow.

As with foot reflexology, scientific research is scanty and mixed, but many people report they find this therapy eases pain and promotes relaxation.

Reiki

This Japanese-based energy therapy was developed in the 19th century by Dr. Mikao Usui, although it is part of an ancient tradition with roots in ancient India. Reiki draws on the "universal life energy" which is believed to be within each one of us and to exist throughout the world around us. This energy is the same as the *qi* used in Traditional Chinese Medicine (*see The power of* qi, *pages 78–81*).

This universal energy is "channelled" through a Reiki practitioner to areas in a patient's body where it is said to have a healing effect. The theory is that the energy has the power to clear a person's blocked energy when it has contributed to disease and help promote health and well-being.

Reiki practitioners attune themselves so that they can open a healing channel to the universal life energy. In a Reiki session, the therapist places their hands on, or just above, specific places on the patient's body that correspond to energy centres.

Heat-sensitive photographs have shown that the hands of a therapist do indeed become warmer while they are giving a treatment. There is little other objective evidence to support Reiki claims. However, some people say they feel relaxed or invigorated after a Reiki session.

MAGNETS

Magnet therapy goes back to ancient times, when lodestones were believed to contribute to beauty and health. In recent years, magnets in various shapes and sizes have been vigorously promoted for arthritis and other pain relief. They come in wraps, pads and belts for various body parts as well as embedded in jewellery, shoe insoles, pillows and mattresses.

The evidence for static magnets is scanty but they are probably not harmful. In one study, magnetic shoe inserts helped relieve a painful foot condition, and there were mixed results from a study of magnetic mattress pads used for women with fibromyalgia.

There are some studies that show bone-healing and pain-relief benefits from pulsed electromagnetic therapy, in which a mild electric current is passed via magnets through to the body.

Movement therapies

Next to pain, the symptom that most affects people with arthritis is the loss of mobility. Joints and muscles can become stiff and pain may make you reluctant to move, which can lead to yet more stiffness. It is difficult to exercise when you are hurting. The following movement therapies can be adjusted to your level of ability and can help you to retain or regain mobility.

Yoga

Most people think of yoga as a series of stretching exercises, but it is much more than that. Developed thousands of years ago in India to integrate physical, mental and spiritual well-being, the very word

in ancient Sanskrit means "union". Different branches of yoga emphasize different parts of that union. Hatha yoga – a series of gentle stretching exercises and breathing – is the one best known to Westerners.

In hatha yoga, you assume and hold poses called *asanas* that have been designed to develop and balance body and mind, and to stimulate the internal organs and nerves. These can be done by people of any age and, with adaptation, just about any level of fitness or disability. Practitioners work

PRACTISING TAI CHI
No matter what their age or ability, Chinese people gather together outside on a regular daily basis to practise the sequences of tai chi.

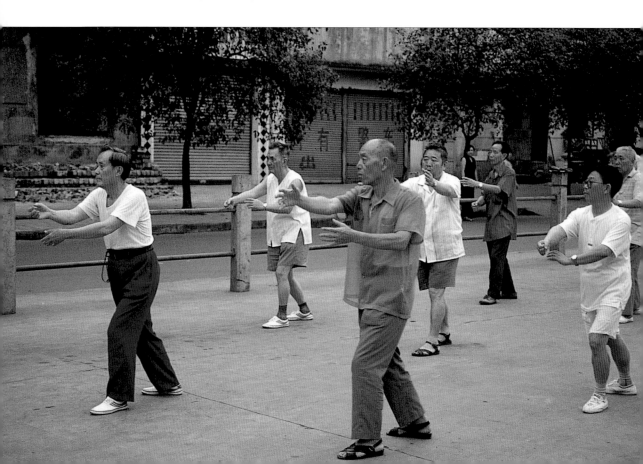

within individual limits – perfection in attaining the exact pose is not as important as the process. Many yoga classes end with deep relaxation and/or meditation.

For people with arthritis, yoga can have many rewards. Studies show it can improve arthritis of the hands and contribute to energy levels and relaxation. Yoga is known to improve flexibility, strength and mental and physical balance. Practised daily, it can contribute significantly to your health. Many people report feeling calm and relaxed after yoga.

Yoga is best learned in a class, from an instructor experienced in working with your type of arthritis who can recommend the best *asanas* for you. Beware of instructors or classes that emphasize the exercise aspects of yoga and make sure the class you choose is safe for people with arthritis. If your arthritis is very severe or disabling, ask for a referral to a yoga instructor who is also a physiotherapist or who has had special training.

Tai chi and qigong

The gentle and powerful movements of tai chi have many healing advantages that can be very beneficial to people with arthritis and other musculoskeletal conditions (*see Chapters 4, 5 and 6*).

Qigong is closely related to tai chi and is part of Traditional Chinese Medicine. It is an ancient system of movement and breathing exercises that have been developed to strengthen the body and balance the flow of life energy, or *qi* (*see Chapters 4 and 6*).

MOVEMENT RE-EDUCATION

Our bodies were made for moving. But we may acquire inefficient and even harmful ways of holding and moving the body, especially if there is pain or stiffness from arthritis.

Bad habits can contribute to more joint damage. Studies show that people who are bow-legged or knock-kneed are at increased risk from OA of the knee.

Movement re-education programmes can increase body awareness and help you find less painful ways to use your body. They may also help after joint replacement surgery. Both the following programmes require you to commit time and effort, but the rewards can include better balance and flexibility, and less pain and stress.

FELDENKRAIS METHOD

This was developed by physicist, engineer and athlete Moshe Feldenkrais after he injured his knee. It is based on his theories that certain postures and movements disrupt the nervous system. Taught in classes called "awareness through movement", students begin with very gentle movements, learning how it feels to move and be without pain or discomfort. There are also one-on-one sessions that involve gentle manipulation.

ALEXANDER TECHNIQUE

This was developed by actor Mathias Alexander when he recognized that vocal and throat problems were related to tension and stress in the way he held his body. The technique, which is usually taught one-on-one, teaches people how to recognize their postural problems and to stand and move with more ease.

Herbs & homeopathy

Modern drugs can be life-saving for acute ailments and can slow or stop the progress of joint-damaging inflammation. But they can have strong side effects, especially when taken daily for many years. Concern about side effects is one reason some people with arthritis have looked to "natural" remedies, such as herbs and homeopathic treatments.

Herbs and medicinal plants

Most medicinal plants haven't been studied scientifically for their effect on arthritis, but evidence suggests some might help relieve pain and inflammation. Among herbs and spices that show promise are green tea, ginger, flaxseed and turmeric (*see Healing foods, pages 28–31*). Herbal remedies are available in many forms, including capsules,

tablets, tinctures (herbs steeped in alcohol), lotions, ointments, teas or poultices.

Below are some medicinal plants that have been shown to help with arthritis symptoms. Others include St John's wort for depression, valerian for improving sleep quality and easing anxiety, and kava kava for relaxing and easing anxiety.

Boswellia, ginger and turmeric

These plants can block inflammation and have been shown, in a combination product with the Indian herb ashwagandha, to ease symptoms of OA and RA.

Boswellia is frankincense, a gummy substance usually taken in pill form. Ginger (*see page 29*) can be eaten with many foods, made into a tea by steeping a teaspoon of fresh grated ginger in a cup of warm water or taken in tincture, capsule or tablet form. Turmeric (*see page 31*), an Asian spice used in curries, also comes in tablets and capsules. **Caution:** ginger is a blood-thinner so take care when using it with other blood-thinners (*see page 53*).

GLA oils

The oils from evening primrose, borage and blackcurrant contain gamma linolenic acid (GLA), an omega-6 fatty acid that our body uses to make anti-inflammatory chemicals. Studies show that GLA oil supplements can ease inflammation and pain from RA. GLA is available in capsules and cold-pressed oils. The usual dosage is about 1,800mg of GLA per day. **Caution:** GLAs are blood-thinners (*see page 53*).

TAKE WITH CAUTION

Herbs and medicinal plants appeal to many because they are "natural." But just because something is natural doesn't mean it's safe. Anything strong enough to help is strong enough to hurt. Herbs can have side effects as well as modern medicines and few have been carefully studied yet for safety or effectiveness

Check labels or consult a herbalist for the appropriate herb or dosage for your individual situation. Dosages given here are approximate: your safe and effective dose may be different, depending on your body weight and other factors, including the effects of other drugs or herbs you maybe taking. Do not use herbs if you are pregnant or nursing.

Stinging nettle

An ancient remedy for arthritis, test–tube studies have shown nettle leaf extract blocked inflammatory chemicals. In one study, 50mg of an extract enhanced the effects of the anti–inflammatory drug diclofenac for people with OA, allowing them to reduce their NSAID dosage. Nettle leaves can be stewed and eaten, or extracts taken in capsules. Check labels for dosage.

Homeopathy

Homeopathy is based on the idea that "like cures like," and that very diluted amounts of a poison or other disease–causing substance can stimulate the body to relieve the same symptoms that the larger dose causes. Although many people use homeopathy there is no hard scientific evidence to prove the remedies have an effect on arthritis.

A homeopath will examine you and talk about your symptoms and then select the remedies for your specific situation. Often, a single remedy is tried.

The remedies are usually made from plants and minerals and are so diluted – often not a single molecule of the "active" ingredient remains – they are unlikely to cause harm. Remedies can be bought off the shelf, labelled with the condition they are usually used to treat.

Among homeopathic remedies used for for arthritis pain are *Rhus Tox* (poison ivy); *Byronia* (wild hops); *Apis* (crushed bees); *Ledum* (wild rosemary); and *Aurum metallicum* (gold). For gout *Colchicum autumnale* (meadow saffron) is used.

AROMATHERAPY

The essential oils of aromatherapy can affect your physical, emotional and spiritual levels, helping to relax you and relieve tension.

Scents may provoke a powerful emotional and physical reaction, bringing back memories and affecting our mood. The olfactory system controlling the sense of smell is closely linked to the hypothalamus, the part of our brain concerned with mood and emotions. There is evidence that inhaled essential oils affect brain waves and that some scents may relieve anxiety and ease stress.

The power of scent has been used in many cultures to treat illness and promote health and beauty. Aromatherapy practice has connected the smells of essential oils taken from trees, flowers and roots with certain properties and effects. Lavender, for example, is said to be a good sedative and an effective antidepressant; and chamomile is thought to have anti-inflammatory properties.

In aromatherapy, the essential oils are added to baths, diluted with other oils and used for massage or evaporated in oil burners to scent a room.

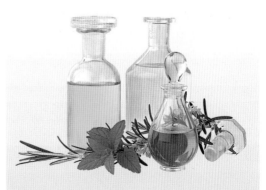

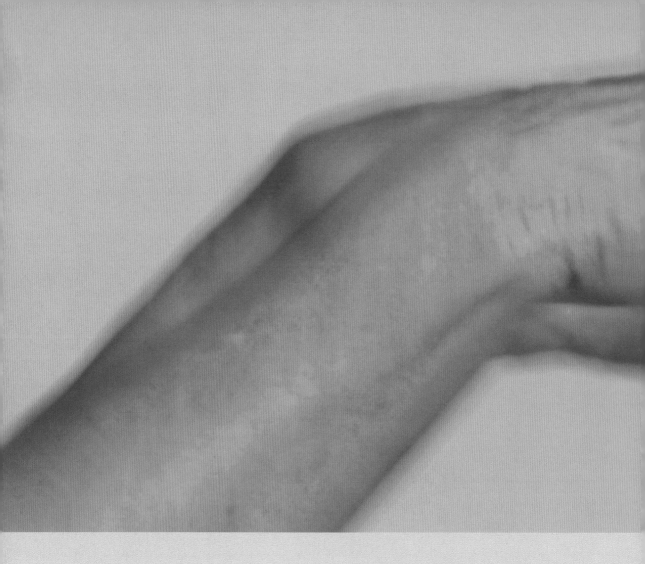

The healing power
of tai chi

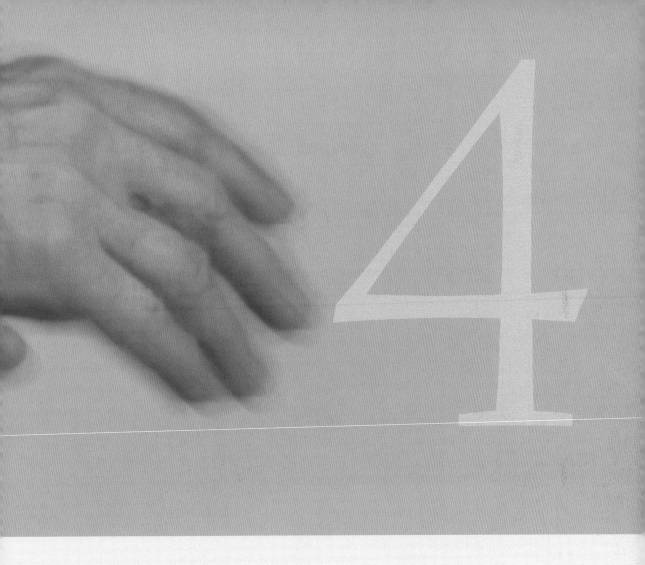

Tai chi is a remarkable system of exercises that can break through the vicious circle of symptoms that characterize arthritis. Tai chi movements will help to relieve pain, stiffness and stress and so improve flexibility, balance and coordination.

What is tai chi?

Every day, hundreds of millions of people around the world practise tai chi, a traditional Chinese movement programme designed to integrate the body, mind and spirit. Tai chi is an exercise and method of self–defence as well as an art form and a relaxation technique. It has been described as part martial art, part exercise and part meditation.

Tai chi is composed of a series of gentle, graceful movements linked together in a continuous, smooth–flowing sequence. Each tai chi movement is precisely choreographed to flow rhythmically into the next, moving the body through a coordinated sequence during which the mind stays relaxed yet focused. There are many styles of tai chi and each style has its own set of sequences called a form.

Often called "meditation in motion", tai chi is performed with total concentration and inner stillness. This inner calm within the movement improves the flow of *qi* (pronounced "chee"), the vital life energy that Chinese philosophy believes sustains and improves health.

Tai chi relies not on outer physical strength but on inner awareness to achieve balance and provides the mental relaxation, physical fitness and spiritual balance so essential to our modern stress-filled lives. This union of the physical, mental and spiritual can provide many benefits in all aspects of life. With regular practice, tai chi can increase flexibility, build strength, improve balance and coordination, enhance the immune system and improve concentration and memory.

Tai chi can be pleasing to do, easy to learn and may be practised almost anywhere. It is used by people of all ages to relieve pain, stress and anxiety, and to promote inner peace. The upright posture aligns the spine; the deep diaphragmatic breathing nourishes and relaxes muscles and spirit; and the slow motions take most of your joints and muscles gently through their complete range of movement.

The martial arts connection

You may not be interested in the martial art aspects of tai chi. Indeed, the practise of martial art tai chi is not recommended for most people with arthritis. But it will help you to understand the internal component of tai chi movements if you know what the movements were intended to achieve. Tai chi's philosophical approach to self–defence can help you mentally gain control of your arthritis.

You may know of martial arts that feature vigorous body movements, dynamic kicks and harsh punching actions. By contrast, tai chi is made up of fluid, graceful and circular movements that come from an internal awareness. You seem to yield to the opponent's force while, at the same time, gaining an understanding of the attack, and then taking control and redirecting it away from you.

Arthritis is described as "attacking" the joints and people with arthritis can feel they have to "fight" their condition. But returning aggression with aggression will not help you conquer the problem.

Practising tai chi means that you don't waste energy "fighting" the diagnosis with anger, denial and depression, or focusing on the effects of your disease. Rather, you will learn as much as possible about this "opponent" and then use your physical, mental and spiritual energies in the best way to protect your health.

The power of *qi*

To understand tai chi, it is useful to know something about the principles and practice of Chinese medicine, a 2,000-year-old healing tradition which is still widely used throughout China today and is becoming increasingly popular in the West.

The essential principles of Traditional Chinese Medicine are based on ancient Taoist philosophy, which stresses the natural balance in all things and encourages the need for people to live in spiritual and physical accord with the patterns of nature.

The overall aim of Traditional Chinese Medicine is to help you prevent disease by living in balance and harmony, which leads naturally to better health and a longer life. When you are out of harmony, disease and discomfort result.

Being in harmony means balancing the complementary polarities of *yin* and *yang* (*see page 80*) and balancing the flow of *qi* in the body. These concepts are at the heart of Traditional Chinese Medicine.

Qi is difficult to translate. You cannot see or measure *qi*. It means "air" and vital life energy. But it also means much more than that. It is life itself, an invisible force that is in every living thing.

The importance of *qi* for health

Qi flows through all parts of our bodies in about a dozen invisible channels called meridians (which have no counterpart in Western anatomy). It is believed that *qi* contributes to many functions that maintain energy and good health.

The stronger *qi* you have, the healthier and stronger you are. When *qi* flows through the body smoothly and powerfully, it will enhance and bring about healing.

Each of us is born with a certain amount of *qi* that we inherit from our parents. We continue to take in more *qi* through the air we breathe, through our food and drink, and through meditation and exercise systems, such as tai chi and qigong (*see page 80*).

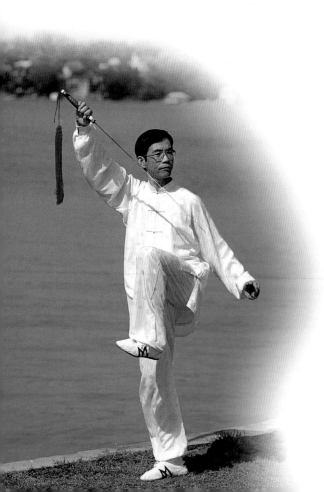

TAI CHI SWORD
The sword is a beautiful extension of tai chi, more suitable for advanced practitioners.

Traditional Chinese Medicine helps balance *yin* and *yang* and improves the flow of *qi* in the body. To achieve this, practitioners use acupuncture, acupressure, tai chi, qigong, herbal medicine and massage.

When the flow of *qi* through your body is blocked or unbalanced, illness results. Illness may also block the flow of *qi*. In Chinese medicine, treatments are aimed at helping each individual maintain balance by unblocking or strengthening the flow of *qi* through proper exercise, herbal medicine, diet and stress management.

According to Chinese medicine, arthritis is caused by weak and sluggish flow of *qi* in the body. For centuries Chinese doctors have recommended tai chi for people with arthritis because it is a very effective way of cultivating strong *qi*.

THE ADVANTAGES OF TAI CHI

Tai chi is one of the most attractive exercise programmes because:

- Almost anyone can do tai chi, whatever your age or physical condition.
- You don't need any expensive equipment, which means you can do it just about anywhere, either outdoors or inside.
- You can do it either alone or in a group.
- It's easy to learn and do. Within weeks of regular practice, you will find your health and well-being have improved.
- You will find it easy to practise regularly on a daily basis. It's enjoyable and you will find 10 or 20 minutes a day to practise.
- The more you progress, the more you can learn. Some compare it to peeling an onion: there is layer inside layer inside layer.

THE MEDICAL BENEFITS OF TAI CHI AND QIGONG

Doctors in China have long recommended tai chi and qigong as a preventive and therapy for many ailments. These practices have been shown to help with pain and other symptoms and to contribute to a better quality of life for people with the following:

- Rheumatoid arthritis
- Osteoarthritis (degenerative joint disease)
- Fibromyalgia
- Ankylosing spondylitis
- Osteoporosis
- Chronic pain
- Chronic fatigue syndrome
- Heart disease
- High blood pressure (hypertension)

- Stress, anxiety
- Diabetes
- Depression
- Rehabilitation from surgery, serious illness and injuries
- Multiple sclerosis

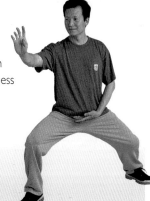

Feeling your own *qi*

As you practise tai chi or qigong, you may find it difficult at first to perceive your *qi*. Don't worry: even if you cannot consciously feel your *qi*, the method will still deliver health benefits. After some practice, it will come to you. You will develop your own awareness of *qi*, though you may describe it differently from others. You may experience *qi* as a magnetic force between your hands, or as a warmth or tingling in your hands.

Many people feel *qi* as a pleasant, warm and slightly heavy feeling. Others sense it as a deep wave of calm energy through their entire body. As you practise you may feel as though you are enclosed in warm energy, and that your body, mind and spirit are more "settled" and stable, relaxed but alert.

Qigong

This ancient practice involves breathing, meditation and movement exercises. There are many styles, from a "still", or meditative, exercise with little or no movement to a more vigorous, athletic form. Meditative qigong can be done by anyone, even those who are bedridden. The simpler forms of moving qigong are very easy for people with arthritis (*see pages 132–35*).

Individual qigong practice can improve or maintain health. It is believed that some qigong masters can channel and direct their *qi* towards other people to help them heal. Researchers believe a major benefit of qigong lies in the way it helps to regulate the nervous system and brain function, contributing to stress relief and relaxation.

YIN, YANG AND TAI CHI

According to Chinese philosophy everything in nature is composed of two opposite but complementary elements called yin *and* yang. *Together, they represent the elements within nature, forever changing yet always in a state of harmony and balance.*

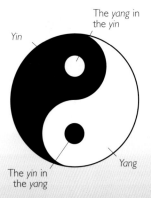

The *yang* in the *yin*

Yin

The *yin* in the *yang*

Yang

Yin is the feminine element: it is softer, more pliant, passive and more negative. *Yang* is masculine: harder, more rigid, active and more positive. Nothing is ever completely *yin* and nothing completely *yang*. The seed of one is found in the heart of the other.

Both *yin* and *yang* complement each other fully and together form a perfect whole. The traditional symbol for *yin* and *yang* (*left*) shows how intertwined and cyclic they are. This symbol, by the way, is also used as a representation of tai chi.

Tai chi means "the ultimate of ultimate" and comes from the 3,000-year-old Book of Changes (*I Ching*) where it is written that "in every change exists tai chi, which causes the two opposites in everything".

SUN STYLE TAI CHI

The origins of tai chi are controversial, yet it is clear that the sequences were developed with great thoughtfulness and a deep knowledge of the human body and spirit. Each of the many styles of tai chi, such as Sun style, offers a complete work-out for body, mind and spirit.

We believe Sun style is the best tai chi style for arthritis because it contains many deep and powerful qigong exercises that further enhance and balance the flow of *qi*, and enrich your tai chi practice. The gentle and slow movements will open up your energy channels and keep them strong and supple; the rhythmic movements of the muscle, spine and joints will pump energy throughout your whole body; and the deep concentration will quiet and unite your body, mind and spirit.

Sun style is the youngest of the major tai chi styles. It was developed by Sun Lu-tang (1861–1932), a well-known exponent of two famous styles of martial art (called Xingyiquan and Baguaquan). He in his early 50s when he learned to practise tai chi from Hao Weizheng, a famous master.

Sun style tai chi is characterized by a high stance and agile steps. Whenever one foot moves forwards or backwards, the other foot follows, so that all movements flow smoothly, like water in a river.

It is deeply beneficial: whenever you turn, there are opening and closing movements that have much healing power. Sun style does not require deep knee bends and is very gentle, making it especially suitable for people with arthritis or other musculoskeletal conditions.

WHY SUN STYLE?

We chose the Sun style of tai chi for people with arthritis and related musculoskeletal conditions for the following reasons:

* It is rich in powerful qigong exercises, which are especially effective for healing and relaxation.
* The higher, more upright, stance of Sun style puts less stress on the knees and hips, and thus makes it more suitable for people with arthritis and for older people.
* The sequences keep you moving. The movements of one foot are followed by the other, so you move more often than in other tai chi styles, and do not over-stress your joints. Increased mobility is well accepted by doctors to be beneficial for people with arthritis.
* The agile movements make it easy to keep one's balance and yet contribute to the improvement of balance.
* The movements are compact, involving few steps, so you do not require a large space in which to practise.
* Sun style can be easy to learn but has so much depth that, even with daily practice, it will hold your interest.

The health benefits of tai chi

Many of us find our lives out of balance today, especially when coping with arthritis and other musculoskeletal conditions. It's a vicious circle: your arthritis causes you pain, which results in stress, which makes all of your symptoms worse, which in turn makes you anxious and depressed, which finally causes you more pain. You can feel out of control with the combination of emotional turmoil and physical pain.

There is no doubt that exercise and relaxation can help all of these symptoms and bring a sense of balance back into your life. Study after study shows that we need to keep moving to be healthy and strong, and that stress and anxiety will contribute to pain, heart disease, stiffness and several other disabilities.

Getting joints in motion

People with arthritis are often not eager to exercise. And no wonder: it's hard to even think about working out when pain and stiffness make it difficult to move at all. Moreover, the wrong kind of exercise can lead to injuries for people with arthritis and musculoskeletal problems and contribute to their symptoms. Tai chi is the right kind of exercise and its health benefits are many (*see box, page 83*).

Numerous scientific studies have shown that tai chi can help ease many of the symptoms connected with arthritis – and that people find tai chi enjoyable. In more than one study, people practising tai chi regularly showed more improvement than those taking other forms of exercise, which may have been because the tai chi students were exercising more. Other studies have also shown that regular tai chi practice is safe for people in frail health, including those with rheumatoid arthritis.

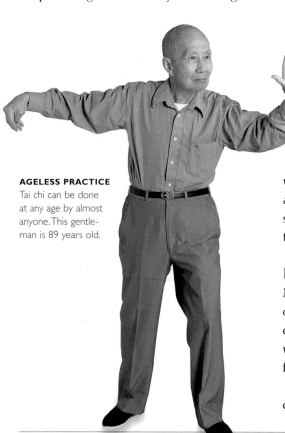

AGELESS PRACTICE
Tai chi can be done at any age by almost anyone. This gentleman is 89 years old.

Improved flexibility and balance

Many studies show that tai chi, either alone or in combination with other treatments, can improve balance and prevent falls, which is especially encouraging evidence for those with arthritis

Stiffness and pain from arthritis can contribute to poor balance. Several studies have shown that regular tai chi practice can significantly increase flexibility, balance and coordination, especially among the elderly. This is particularly good news for older people or for those with osteoporosis who may suffer serious injuries from a fall.

Many people with arthritis have osteoporosis (*see page 55*), a condition in which loss of bone mass makes their bones brittle. Your risk of developing osteoporosis increases if you are taking certain arthritis medications, such as the corticosteroid drug prednisolone, which is often prescribed to help control the symptoms of rheumatoid arthritis or lupus.

The most serious potential damage from osteoporosis is the increased risk of broken bones. In the elderly, fractures can mean the difference between an independent and active life and being bedridden. Tai chi practice, together with drug or hormone therapy, can help to prevent or slow osteoporosis damage by contributing to strong bones and muscles – tai chi is a weight–bearing exercise that is gentle enough even for frail bones.

Other studies have endorsed tai chi's usefulness. In one study in Atlanta in the US in 1996, a 15–week programme of tai chi was found to improve significantly the flexibility, strength and cardiovascular endurance of people who were 70 or older – and to reduce the risk of multiple falls by 47.5 per cent.

In another study in 1987, researchers at the University of Florida found that tai chi enabled those with rheumatoid arthritis to

TAI CHI AS AN EXERCISE AND THERAPY FOR ARTHRITIS

Tai chi is a remarkable system of exercises that not only stimulates the flow of energy throughout the body but also encourages the muscles, bones and joints to carry out the movements for which they were designed. Tai chi removes energy blockages to enhance the flow of qi and helps to integrate mind and body to restore health and well-being. It is known that tai chi:

- Helps to relieve pain and ease stiffness in joints.
- Improves overall balance and physical coordination.
- Improves posture and the way people stand and move.
- Strengthens muscles and builds stamina.
- Increases circulation of the blood and lymph and improves the function of both the heart and lungs.
- Relieves stress, anxiety and depression.
- Improves concentration and memory.

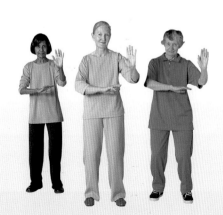

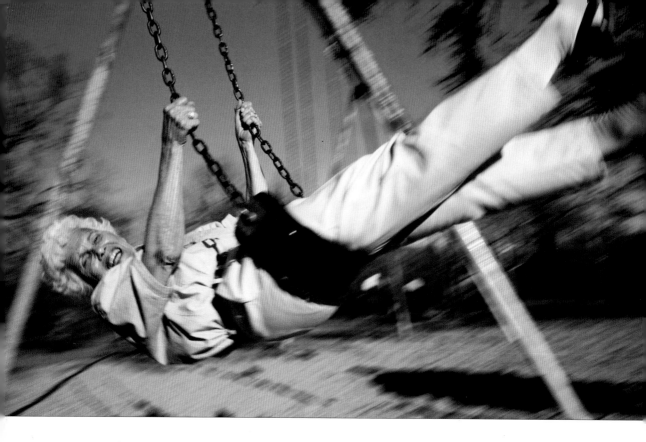

improve the range of motion in their arms
and shoulders – and this benefit continued
for four months after they had finished the
tai chi programme.

Pain relief

Arthritis can be either an uncomfortable
inconvenience or a devastating, disabling
illness. Either way, the symptom people
say affects their lives the most is the pain.

Pain prevents you having a good night's
sleep and taking healthy exercise. It can rob
you of the activities you used to enjoy. At
its worst, chronic pain can isolate you from
friends and family.

Conventional medications prescribed to
control pain all have side effects (*see Chapter
Three*) and may not control pain sufficiently
or ease the stiffness. Practising tai chi
regularly, however, can help to relieve pain

FREEDOM TO ENJOY
Regular tai chi practice breaks the vicious circle of pain,
stress and depression, offering a more active lifestyle and
the freedom to enjoy the benefits of everyday activities.

by exercising your joints, which pumps
fluids into the cartilage; by strengthening
the muscles that hold the joints in place;
and by circulating blood, lymph and other
fluids to promote health.

Tai chi calms the mind and promotes
relaxation which relieves pain and tension.
Tension and stress are known to make
pain worse and to contribute to the flares
(*see page 99*) that are associated with arthritis
and fibromyalgia.

A number of studies support tai chi and
qigong's contribution to pain relief. In 1999,
a pilot study of tai chi for the elderly found
that it helped to improve mood and quality
of life; and, in 2000, a University of Arizona

review of therapies for pain found that tai chi and meditation used with medication could significantly reduce pain.

A study of 28 women with fibromyalgia found that an eight-week programme of qigong practice, combined with mindfulness meditation and techniques for managing pain, gave significant improvement in pain threshold, depression, coping and function. A follow-up study showed that these results persisted for at least four months after the programme had been completed.

Biomechanics and strength

Many doctors and physiotherapists believe our biomechanics – the way we stand and move – can contribute to the risk of arthritis or make it worse. OA, for example, often develops in athletes who regularly injure the same joints and in people whose work puts repeated stress on the same joints.

There are two types of strengthening exercise in tai chi: isometric exercise, in which muscles are tightened but the joints do not move; and isotonic exercise, in which muscles are strengthened by moving the joints. Studies show that these exercises in tai chi can improve posture, balance and efficient movement by preventing stress on joints and muscles, so preventing cartilage wear. In a Taiwan study, tai chi practice significantly eased pain and stiffness and improved function in those with knee OA.

A further benefit is that tai chi's upright, powerful but supple posture contributes to a positive mental attitude. A stooped body is often associated with sadness, fear and negative emotion.

CIRCULATION AND HEART DISEASE

Heart disease is a major cause of death worldwide, and hypertension (high blood pressure) is common in developed countries. People with some kinds of arthritis, such as lupus and RA, or those who take some medications, are at increased risk of heart disease.

Most people accept that regular exercise and deep relaxation help to lower blood pressure and to reduce the risks of heart disease.

Studies have shown that tai chi can lower blood pressure just as well as the more energetic aerobic exercises. Moreover, tai chi has been shown to be more effective than a self-adjusted home exercise programme for low-risk patients who are recovering from heart bypass surgery.

In 2000, a study conducted at the Chinese University of Hong Kong compared the heart rate response and flexibility among two groups of 66-year-old men after a three-minute step test. One group had been practising tai chi for a long time while the other group had been largely inactive.

The group of 28 tai chi practitioners had significantly better scores in both their resting heart rates and their heart rates after the step test. They also scored higher in the flexibility exercises that involved body rotation, reach and the ability to stand on a single leg with their eyes closed.

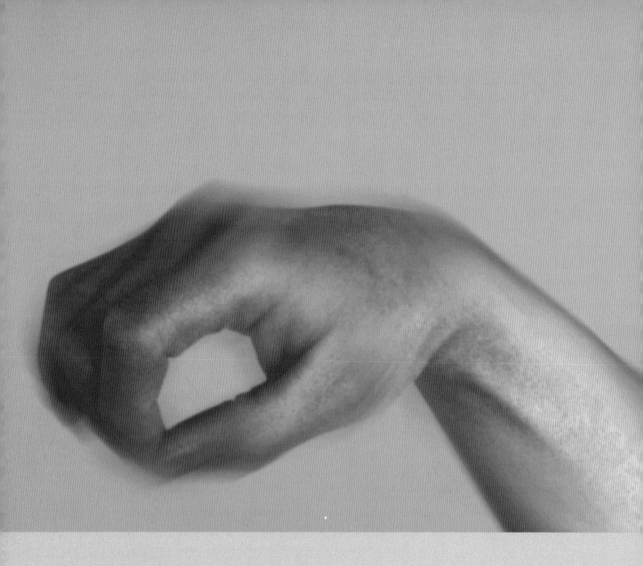

Preparing to do
tai chi

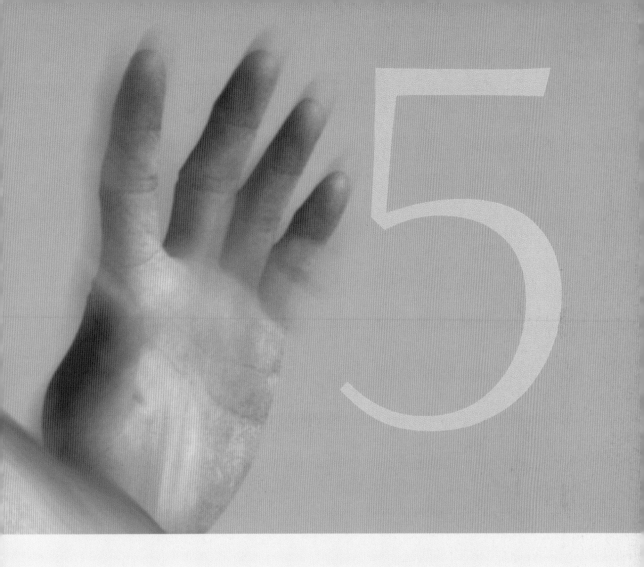

Tai chi is more powerful than it looks. Before you
start make sure you prepare fully. This chapter will
explain how to get the most from your tai chi and
show how breathing, body awareness, meditation
and visualization are essential to your practice.

Tai Chi for Arthritis programme

The Tai Chi for Arthritis programme was designed specifically for people with musculoskeletal conditions by Dr. Paul Lam, a tai chi team and a health team that includes rheumatologists and a physiotherapist (*see page 144*). The Arthritis Foundation of Australia uses the programme and supports the workshops in which Dr. Lam and his team train instructors.

Although all tai chi emphasizes smooth and deliberate movements, some versions are much more athletic than others and may not be suitable for people with arthritis. The programme is simple yet complete, based on the Sun style of tai chi (*see page 81*). It is safe and delivers significant benefits to people with arthritis within a short time. Since the beginning of the Tai Chi for Arthritis programme, thousands of people have found that it has helped them become stronger, feel better and learn to take control of their condition – whatever their individual symptoms may be.

The programme is short and suitable for almost everyone. Its broad benefits include improved flexibility and muscle strength, calmer breathing and a deep sense of relaxation and well-being. There are warming-up and cooling-down exercises, a set of exercises to help you learn tai chi walking, qigong exercises to enhance energy and two tai chi practice programmes – the six Basic Movements and six Advanced Movements (*see Chapter Six*).

This chapter will help you prepare for the programme in Chapter Six. You will find guidelines about what to wear, where and when and how long to practise, how to avoid injuring yourself and how to overcome a variety of difficulties.

How to get the most out of your tai chi practice

Tai chi works on both a physical and a mental level. Most of us know about physical fitness: we have all done walking, running or some kind of sport or activity. But you may be unfamiliar with the internal concentration involved in tai chi that makes the physical activity more effective. Tai chi trains us to integrate body, mind and spirit in a powerful practice for health and fitness.

However, you don't need to pay attention to all of these concepts all at once. It takes many years to master all of the mental and physical aspects of tai chi. It is better to progress slowly, becoming more aware of your body, feeling your *qi* and beginning to "taste" and enjoy the movements.

Work on one thing at a time for a few days before moving on to the next. Then you can begin to put the bits together. Be patient. Be happy with anything you achieve; praise yourself for any progression and avoid getting frustrated. Remember, it is the tai chi way to "go with the flow of nature" and to enjoy the process and the journey.

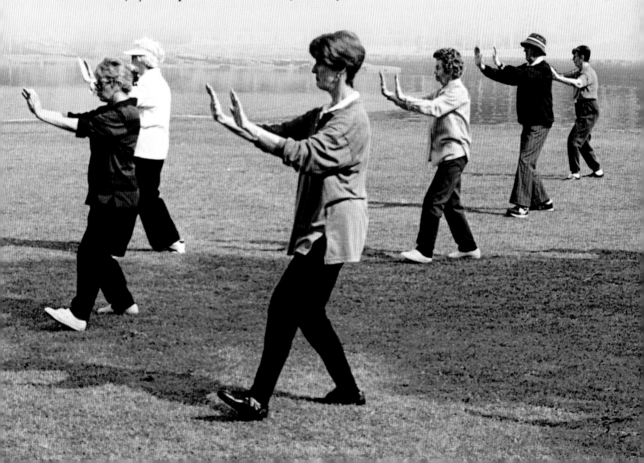

Getting ready to practise

Before you begin to learn the movements of tai chi, find a space where you can move freely and plan a practice time when you will not be distracted or hurried. Decide how long you are going to practise and familiarize yourself with the guidelines for what to do when you are in pain and how to avoid injury.

What to wear

As a general rule, wear comfortable clothes and supportive shoes.

Clothing

You don't need any special clothing for tai chi, but do be sure to wear something loose that will not interfere with either your movements or your circulation. Don't wear tights, leotards or other stretch workout clothes. Track suits or light trousers with an elastic waist are good, along with a T-shirt or loose-knit shirt. If it is very warm, you can wear shorts.

Shoes

You should wear shoes, both to protect your feet and to offer some stability. Shoes should be flat. Many people prefer shoes especially made for martial arts, which are both lightweight and flat. Other people prefer running shoes or traditional Chinese cloth shoes.

If you need, or are accustomed to wearing, special shoes, orthotics or insoles to correct your balance or gait, then please use them for tai chi. Basically, you should wear shoes that feel comfortable, give you support and

AVOIDING PAIN

You will find your strength increases with regular practice, but don't overdo it. Here are some guidelines for avoiding pain:

- Only practise tai chi for as long as you can easily walk.
- Always stop immediately if any part of your body hurts.
- If pain persists, or if you are suffering some discomfort for more than two hours after a tai chi session, then you are probably doing too much.
- Remember: it is not a competition. Do only what is comfortable for you.

allow you to move and stand with confidence and balance.

Where to practise

The advantage of tai chi is that it can be done almost anywhere since it does not require much space or any special equipment. Any place that is quiet, well-ventilated and has enough room for you to move easily will be fine. Many people prefer to practise outside. Choose a place that is quiet, dry and protected from the wind and direct sun.

When to practise

Set aside the same time every day to work on your tai chi so that it becomes a good habit like cleaning your teeth. In China, you will see hundreds of people gathering in parks early in the morning to practise tai chi before they begin their day. But any time of day is good, as long as you have not just eaten or are not too hungry or tired.

How long to practise

It is important to practise to your ability and within your individual limits – the exact length of time is not so relevant. As a general rule, practise tai chi only as long as you can walk without pain or stress. For example, if you can walk comfortably for half an hour at a time, then practise tai chi for half an hour. However, if your arthritis is more severe and you can only walk for five minutes, then practise for five minutes. After resting for a few minutes, you might be able to resume practice, but don't push too hard.

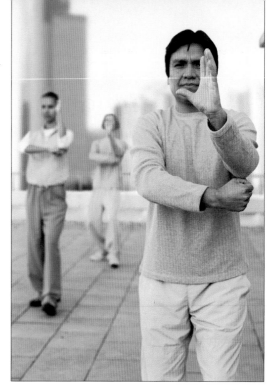

TAI CHI IN A GROUP
One of the advantages of tai chi is that you can learn it with others in a supportive group. You can also practise it outside and you don't need any special equipment.

HOW TO AVOID INJURY

People with joint or muscle problems need to take special care with any exercise. Here are some guidelines for avoiding injury when doing tai chi:

- Don't lock your knees. Keep your knees aligned over your feet, but slightly bent.
- Don't bend your knees too much. If you can't see your toes when you look down, you are bending too deeply (see page 106).
- Don't lean backwards or forwards. Keep your back upright so your spine is balanced over your pelvis.
- Don't force any movement. You should move without effort, as though you were gently swimming in air.
- Avoid any abrupt movements. These will create tension that can put you off balance or injure your muscles. All the movements in the Tai Chi for Arthritis programme are smooth and slow.
- Be careful about twisting your knees. If a tai chi movement calls for you to turn your knees sideways, then do this very slowly and carefully.
- Feel free to modify movements that are uncomfortable for you. Tai chi should be pleasant and enjoyable to do and not an endurance contest.

Abdominal breathing

Breathing is vital. We can do without food and even water for a while, but we cannot go even a few minutes without breathing. Yet many of us don't breathe correctly. We take shallow, short breaths, or even hold our breath sometimes, which contributes to tension and pain.

The breathing technique

Tai chi breathing uses all parts of the lungs, nourishes the body and massages the internal organs. It puts gentle pressure on your heart, stomach and intestines. Deep breathing helps to focus attention, build energy, promote relaxation and control pain. It is a vital part of yoga and is used in childbirth to reduce pain and by athletes to improve their performance.

Breathing is not a conscious process (you cannot stop yourself from breathing) and is controlled by the respiratory centre in the brain. This ensures that you inhale oxygen and expel carbon dioxide. But we can control both the speed of our breathing and the depth of the breaths we take. We can also synchronize our breathing with the movements of our body.

Many of the movements in the Tai Chi for Arthritis programme will require you to breathe in (the in-breath) or breathe out (the out-breath) at the same time as moving your arms or your feet. This is all part of the process of enhancing the *qi* within you, for every time you breathe in you are bringing *qi* into your body and, with it, tremendous benefits for your health.

How to do abdominal breathing

The technique used for tai chi and qigong is known as abdominal, or diaphragmatic, breathing. You will find this nourishing and open way of breathing will carry over into, and benefit other parts of your life.

Most people are in the habit of using only part of their lungs and they seldom let their abdomen "stick out" by allowing it to expand. Abdominal breathing uses all parts of the respiratory system.

BREATHING EXERCISE
One way of doing abdominal breathing is to lie on your back and relax your whole body. Breathe gently through your nose and draw air into your lungs. Feel your abdomen rise as you breathe in and fall as you breathe out.

Begin by lightly touching your upper palate with the tongue. As you breathe in through your nose, imagine that air is travelling through your nose, down the airways to fill the lungs and then the abdomen, making it bulge gently outwards. As you breathe out, the abdomen contracts and you mentally picture the air being squeezed out from your abdomen, lungs, airways and finally out through your nose.

Continue to breathe, but don't force it or try to take huge breaths. You may feel the urge to yawn: that's good, because it allows you to take in even more air. You can use abdominal breathing to calm yourself when you are tense or anxious, and to ease pain.

Tai chi and qigong breathing

As you do tai chi, your breathing should be slow, even, continuous and in rhythm with your movements. But don't force it: you can return to a normal way of breathing at any time. Check often to make sure you are not holding your breath when you are doing tai chi and qigong.

Reverse abdominal breathing

This more advanced technique that allows your *qi* energy to quickly reach your *dan tian* (*see page 94*). As before, imagine the air travelling down the airways to fill your abdomen. But this time let your in-breath expand the upper part of the abdomen (where the stomach is) while your lower abdomen contracts. When you breathe out, the upper abdomen flattens and the lower abdomen extends outwards.

BREATHING DURING TAI CHI PRACTICE

Coordinating your breathing with the movements of your hands, arms and feet is an essential part of tai chi. Here are some general rules:

YOU BREATHE IN WHEN:

- You are bringing your hands closer to your body – for example, at the first part of each repetition of Waving Hands in the Clouds, when you bring your right hand and foot closer to the left (*see page 118, Step 1*).
- You are moving your hands upwards – for example, during the Beginning movement (*see page 114, Step 2*).
- You are pulling your hands apart in a qigong exercise – for example, in Opening & Closing Hands (*see page 116, Step 2*).

YOU BREATHE OUT WHEN:

- You make opening up movements – for example, doing the last part of the third movement, Single Whip, when you stretch out both your hands (*see page 117, Step 3*).
- You are moving your hands downwards (*see page 115, Step 3*).
- You are moving your hands towards each other in a qigong exercise – for example, in Opening & Closing Hands (*see page 116, Step 3*).

Body awareness

Body awareness helps you to coordinate your movements and move with more confidence. It means being aware of where your body is in your environment, in relationship to other people and to objects. This awareness also means knowing which part of your body is carrying pain, what areas need special care and how to find and relax areas of tension.

Because tai chi is a type of martial art, it emphasizes awareness of the body. It was created and developed to sharpen spatial awareness and to show people how to hold their bodies in an alert but relaxed readiness, poised to move in any direction.

As you prepare to do tai chi, explore your joints with your mind. Allow them to become loose and open, not locked and tight. Keep just enough muscle tension to hold them in place, but not so much you cause them to be stiff. This will allow *qi* to flow freely and will also allow your muscles, joints and ligaments to benefit more from the strength–building exercises of the tai chi movements.

One way to find out if you are tense is to check your shoulders. If they're hunched up or forwards, you are carrying tension there. Stretching your shoulders gently outwards and downwards will help them to be loose and open.

Standing and moving

It is very important to keep your back upright when doing tai chi. Many people tend to lean either backwards or forwards, which puts them off balance and can cause strain to muscles and joints. It is especially important to bear this in mind if you have arthritis in the back, hips and knees.

To line up your body, imagine a straight line drawn down through your ear to your

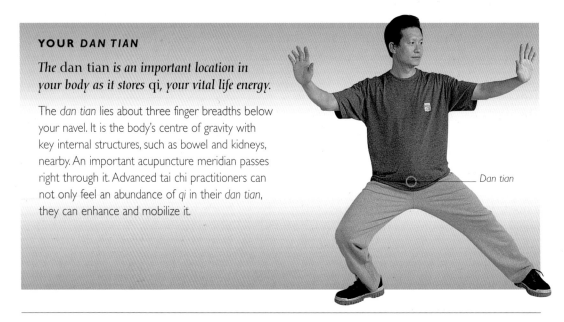

YOUR *DAN TIAN*

The dan tian *is an important location in your body as it stores* qi, *your vital life energy.*

The *dan tian* lies about three finger breadths below your navel. It is the body's centre of gravity with key internal structures, such as bowel and kidneys, nearby. An important acupuncture meridian passes right through it. Advanced tai chi practitioners can not only feel an abundance of *qi* in their *dan tian*, they can enhance and mobilize it.

Dan tian

shoulder, hip and heel. Now imagine a string going up from the crown of your head, gently pulling you upright. When bending your knees be careful not to do too much: imagine another line going through your kneecap to the tip of your toes. If you cannot see your toes when looking down, you are bending your knees too much.

When you are beginning to do tai chi, ask someone to check you or use a mirror to examine your posture from the side. If you don't have a large mirror, try standing near a window so that you can see your reflection and check your posture. Mentally remind yourself to check your posture often when you are doing tai chi.

Moving from your centre

The *dan tian* in your pelvic area (*see box, page 94*) is the foundation for your posture and your centre of balance, both physically and spiritually. For the best balance, you need to feel that your upper body is centred firmly yet flexibly into your pelvic area.

All movements are focused, deliberate and come from this foundation. When you move your hands and arms, imagine they're moving from your centre, not just from your wrists or shoulder. This will help you to keep your shoulders relaxed and your body centred.

Try to do your tai chi movements slowly, smoothly and continuously. You may feel jerky or unsteady at first. It helps if you coordinate movements with breathing, to feel the "flow" in your tai chi. Keep at it: with practice it will become easier.

FOOT POSITIONS

The slow and precise movements of tai chi require you to place your feet very carefully in specific positions. This helps you keep your balance and enables you to shift balance easily.

When beginning a tai chi form, the feet are always close together, representing the unity and balance of *yin* and *yang* (see page 80). The feet move apart during the forms to represent *yin* and *yang* separately.

In each movement, the leg that holds more of the weight is *yang* and the other leg is *yin*. Thus, as your weight is transferred between your feet, the elements of *yin* and *yang* change place, but remain balanced.

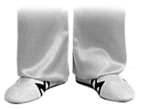

THE UNITY OF *YIN* AND *YANG*
In the first step of each tai chi movement your feet are close together. Think of them as *yin* and *yang*, balanced and unified.

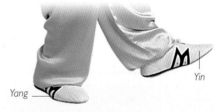

Yang ⎯ Yin

THE SEPARATION OF *YIN* AND *YANG*
During the course of a tai chi movement the feet step apart and *yin* and *yang* temporarily seem to separate. The foot bearing the weight is *yang*, the other foot is *yin*.

Meditation in motion

Most of us live busy lives. We spend little time in the natural world and have lost some of the connection between the conscious mind and the body. You know this when you catch sight of yourself in a mirror or watch a video of yourself in motion and notice your body is not doing exactly what you thought it was. When doing tai chi, for example, you may think your spine is vertical but you are probably leaning slightly.

Habit affects the way we move. All too often, we do things on automatic pilot while our mind is somewhere else. People with painful arthritis of the knee or hip may take pain relievers, and even have a total joint replacement, and yet still move with stiffness or a limp because the mind and body remember the old way of moving.

Training the mind

When beginning a new way of moving and being, you need to train the mind as well as the body. Tai chi is perfect for this, since it helps you learn to cleanse your mind.

Before you begin your tai chi, sit or stand quietly for while. Concentrate on your breath flowing in and out. Allow your abdomen to expand gently with each breath and feel yourself settle down into your abdomen. Now allow your thoughts and worries to flow out with each out-breath. As you breathe in, allow light to fill your head, airways, lungs and abdomen. Take a few deep abdominal breaths (*see page 92–93*).

Tai chi also helps you to focus. As you stand ready to begin tai chi, focus your mind completely to the moment and to yourself in the moment. Concentrate on each movement as you perform it. Don't think ahead to the next step. Just focus on the moment and the sensations of the movements, so that your mind and body are working in harmony.

If your mind starts to wander, bring it gently back to focus on the movement. If pain interrupts you, don't ignore it: adjust your position to be comfortable and then return your focus. Don't let concerns about how "well" you are doing overwhelm you. No one expects you to be an expert right away. With practice and full attention, you will soon be doing tai chi well.

Meditation

For many people, tai chi is a meditative practice that raises consciousness to a higher level of inner peacefulness and oneness with nature. The practice clarifies the mind and increases the flow of *qi*, the vital life energy in all of us.

Tai chi is often called "meditation in motion" because it uses many of the same techniques as meditation and yields similar benefits. The deep breathing, concentration and mindful focus on the movement and the moment restore body, mind and spirit. Like meditation, tai chi can help you find inner calm and put pain, anxiety and stress in perspective. With regular practice, you will find that tension, anger and pain fade into the background. For some people, this may be the first time they experience what it feels like to be without tension.

Visualize your goals

Choose a goal for your tai chi practice. You might, for example, want to feel yourself moving more smoothly between postures; or you might really like to be able to bend your knees with less pain. Set yourself a time limit for your goal; for example, decide that you want to achieve painless movement within one year.

Break your goal down into manageable steps; for example, say that in one month you'll be able to keep your knees partly bent without pain for half the movements. Set a time for daily visualization practice, and decide how long you will spend at it: perhaps five or ten minutes a day.

Now find a quiet place and imagine you are doing the six Basic Movements of the programme in as much detail as possible. Imagine your knees are strong and pain-free. Take the same amount of time in your mind as you would in actual practice.

Your subconscious mind doesn't know this is not real, and will imprint this vision in your body. In time, this visualization will help you achieve your goals. It doesn't work for everyone, but almost anyone will see some kind of improvement.

VISUALIZATION

For some people, spirit refers to the unconscious mind, which can be trained with the powerful methods of positive imagery and visualization.

In visualization, you guide yourself through an experience in your mind, imagining it in detail as vividly as if it were happening. Visualization exercises are often used to relieve pain, anxiety and depression, and to improve physical function. They can greatly improve your internal and external tai chi practice, and many other aspects of your life.

Visualization can be especially useful for people with disabilities, or on days when you have a flare (see page 99) and cannot exercise. Research shows that imagining yourself exercising can affect your body even if you don't move at all: when you think of an action, the part of the brain that controls the action becomes active. In one research study athletes who could not work out visualized themselves going through their routines. When they were able to resume activity, they had not lost any ability: in fact, some improved their physical performance after the mental exercises.

THE POWER OF IMAGINATION
Just thinking about an activity, such as cycling, exerts a powerful effect on the body.

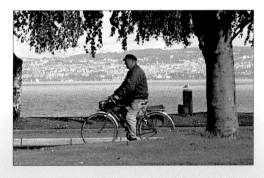

Overcoming difficulties

It is normal to have some discomfort when starting any exercise routine. But you should not feel pain after doing tai chi.

When you first begin tai chi, you may feel some stiffness and mild pain after practice, especially if you have not been very active. But this should disappear within two hours. If not, then you are doing too much – or you need to make some adjustments to your practice. Rest for a day and begin again with a shorter and less demanding session. If you continue to experience pain, please consult your doctor or physiotherapist.

Afterburn

You may find after doing tai chi exercises that you feel a kind of afterburn – your leg muscles or knees are sore, especially if you

have not exercised for a long time or if you have osteoarthritis in the knees. Here are some tips:

• Be careful not to overdo the tai chi exercises at first.

• You can relieve muscle and joint pain with heat and ice. Try soaking a compress in hot Epsom salts and place it on the sore area for 20 minutes or less. Follow this compress with an ice pack – wrap it in fabric so the ice doesn't touch your skin directly – for another 20 minutes or less.

• Elevate your feet while you are sitting down. When lying in bed, lie flat and place a firm pillow under your knees.

• If the pain continues to cause discomfort, you are doing too much. Cut back on the time you exercise and be careful not to bend your knees too much.

PAIN CHECKLIST

Tai chi will help you cultivate body awareness, which in turn can help you relieve or prevent pain. Check the following points as you practise:

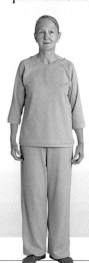

• **Your posture:** are you leaning backwards or forwards? If so, this will strain muscles and joints.

• **Your knees:** are you bending them too far? If your knees are painful, try doing a session without bending them and see how it feels.

• **Your tension:** are your shoulders tight or your arms tense? Tai chi should be done with a relaxed body.

• **Your breathing:** shallow breathing contributes to tension which can cause pain. Tai chi breathing (see *page 93*) is deep, even and coordinated with the movements.

• **Your attitude:** are you trying too hard? Or pushing your body too much? Remember, tai chi for arthritis is not a competitive sport. It is a relaxed and precise way to exercise your body and mind.

Knee and hip pain

Some people with arthritis of the knees and/or the hips may find some tai chi movements are painful or uncomfortable. Check the source: sometimes it is not actually in your knee where you thought it was but in the thigh muscles (quadriceps) that are unaccustomed to exercise. In the same way, pain that appears to be located in your hip may be due to tight hamstring muscles in your legs, or to sore muscles in your lower back.

As you exercise, you will strengthen these muscles, which will then be better at holding your joints in place. But you must build up their strength slowly. Try doing fewer movements at first. Also, try bending your knees less or even straightening up between exercises.

If you have severe arthritis of the knees, you may not be able to bend your knees much at all. Don't worry, that's fine – just do what you can.

After exercise, be sure to do the cooling down movements (*see pages 110–11*). Then you might try a soothing treatment for your knees. You could select one or more of the following: either cold or hot packs (use them separately or alternately); a hot bath, shower or Jacuzzi; pain–relieving ointments or rubs; and massage. You can also try elevating your legs for a few minutes.

Remember: if you experience pain which persists for more than two hours after you have finished your tai chi practice, you are doing too much. Ease off on the amount of time you exercise.

CAUTION

Tai chi can be done safely by virtually anyone, but some movements may not be good for your individual situation. If you are in pain or at all worried about practising tai chi safely, then consult your doctor or physiotherapist first.

When you have flares

A flare is a period of heightened discomfort or pain and is often accompanied by swelling and inflammation. Many things may cause a flare, including emotional or mental stress; physical stress or injury; or an illness such as flu or a cold.

A flare is your body's message to pay attention to the painful part. Respect the message and take special care. Get enough rest and take any prescribed medications. Relaxation and visualization exercises may help reduce the stress (*see pages 96–97*). Cold or hot packs (*see box, page 37*) may ease the pain and swelling.

However, many experts believe you need to keep moving when you have a flare. The idea is that it helps to maintain flexibility and range of motion in your affected joints and muscles, and that it improves blood and fluid circulation throughout your body. Mild exercise also helps you feel better emotionally and more alert mentally. Ask your doctor what is best for you.

But move carefully at all times. Focus attention on each movement, doing it only for as long as it is comfortable. Don't push yourself. Perhaps you can only do the warm-up exercises. Or perhaps you can't bend your knees. That's fine. The important thing is to keep moving.

The basic qigong exercise on pages 132–35 may help you to deal with flares: if you are in great pain try the exercise sitting down. If you cannot move at all, try a visualization (*see page 97*).

Helpful advice on getting going

Tai chi with its gentle circular movements may not seem demanding, but in fact you do quite a lot of work. If your arthritis is severe or painful, you may need some extra help getting going. Here are some strategies:
* Take a warm shower or bath about an hour before to loosen up your muscles. Some people with rheumatoid arthritis may find a cool shower or bath helps more.
* Take a short walk (ten minutes or less) on level ground before and after your tai chi.
* Ask your doctor if you can take a mild pain–relieving drug, such as an over-the-counter medicine, before starting exercise. About half of your usual dose of a pain medication may take the edge off your stiffness so you can move more easily. Be careful not to push through the pain. If the pain persists, consult your doctor.
* Use supports, such as braces, wraps or walkers, when you need them.
* Find a friend to join you in your tai chi practice at least once a week. You may find companionship makes it easier to do your exercise regularly.
* Don't give up: it may take a few weeks to feel the beneficial effects of your tai chi

programme. Commit yourself to a short daily practice for at least six weeks. Keep a diary and note how you feel each day before and after exercising. This will help you see how regular daily exercise can improve the quality of your life.

Tai chi for all abilities

Most people with arthritis have some level of disability. At times, this may be worse, especially when you are having a flare or are under stress. No matter what your physical ability, you can adapt the Tai Chi for Arthritis programme to suit your needs.

Many tai chi students are well into their eighties. Others are young children. Tai chi can be done by people with multiple sclerosis and severe rheumatoid arthritis. If you have difficulty walking or are in a wheelchair, the movements can be adapted to your needs. Even a person who is bedridden can practise some tai chi or qigong exercises.

People often feel that they have to put a big effort into their exercise to get any benefit. That's not true: even a few minutes a day of tai chi, done as best as you can, will benefit you.

If stiffness or pain interferes

You may find that you cannot do the movements as described when you have a flare or even on a good day. Or you may find some movements painful. Whatever you do, don't give up.

First, try the helpful advice on getting going (*see left*). Then look for ways to adapt the movements. For example, if there is stiffness in your elbow and you cannot push your hands as far as the movement requires, extend your hands only as far as is comfortable. At the same time, however, imagine that your arms are completing the movement as directed. Imagining yourself doing tai chi helps to clear and focus your mind while simultaneously relaxing you. It will, over time, actually make it easier for you to do the movements.

If you can't walk or stand easily

Your arthritis may prevent you from walking easily, or from flexing your knee and/or hip joints as much as required. Or you may find you tire easily.

Try doing some of the movements while standing in one place, without bending your knees. Have a walker or chair nearby, in case you need it for support. Just do what you can, within your comfort zone, and then visualize yourself performing the complete movement. Be sure to sit down when you get tired.

If you can move your lower limbs to any extent, simply move what you can and visualize yourself doing the rest of the movements. If you can't walk at all, try doing tai chi while sitting, doing as many movements as you can. You will find that breathing and moving your arms and upper body helps to improve your circulation. If you like, you can just do the upper body movements, especially the qigong breathing exercises (*see pages 132–35*).

Tai chi in your mind

If you cannot move easily at all or if you're having a very painful day, you can do tai chi in your mind. Visualize yourself doing the exercises. Pay attention to details. Ask someone to read the instructions; breathe deeply as you imagine yourself moving.

If you have limited mobility, move as much as you can to follow the programme. Visualize the rest, "seeing" yourself move through the Tai Chi for Arthritis programme (*see page 97*). Studies show that visualizing movements actually has a beneficial effect on the parts of the body you are thinking about.

TAI CHI WHILE SITTING DOWN
People who are unable to stand can still benefit from tai chi – simply do the breathing and upper body movements combined with visualization.

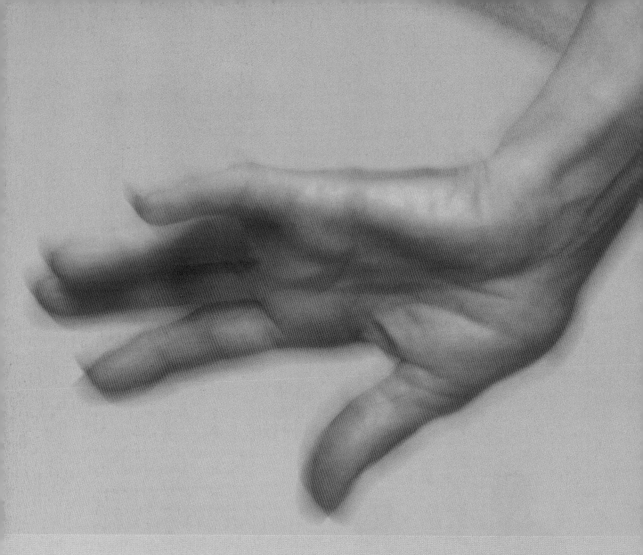

The tai chi
programme

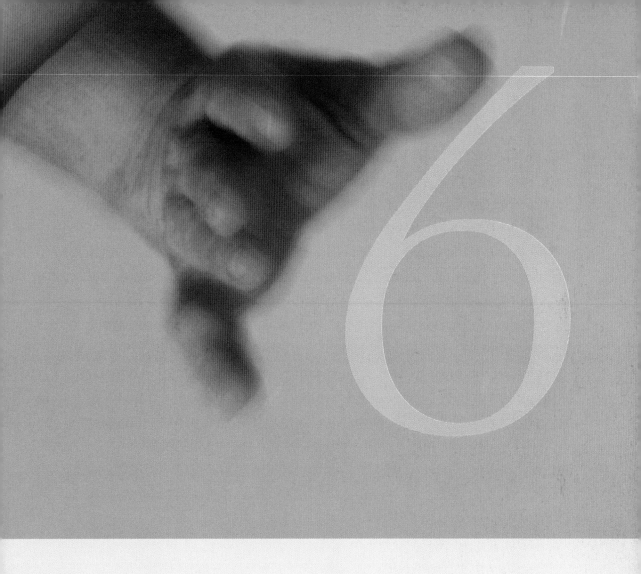

The twelve movements of the Tai Chi for Arthritis programme are safe, straightforward and gentle exercises which Dr. Lam and a team of experts have specifically designed and developed for people with arthritis and other musculoskeletal conditions.

Tai Chi for Arthritis: The Practice

The Tai Chi for Arthritis programme is composed of two carefully chosen sequences: the six Basic Movements (*see pages 114–21*) and the six Advanced Movements (*see pages 122–31*). It also includes a basic but powerful qigong sequence (*see pages 132–35*) to build stamina and improve the flow of energy.

The programme begins with warming-up and cooling-down exercises. Always take the time before each tai chi session to warm up joints and muscles (*see pages 107–9*) and be sure to finish with the cooling-down movements (*see pages 110–11*). Never stop tai chi or any exercise abruptly.

Learn each movement individually and then, when you are confident, move on to the next. As you progress, the tai chi movements will become easier and will flow together in a sequence. Don't rush: take time to become confident with the Basic Movements before moving on to learn the Advanced sequence. If you want to take your tai chi practice further, you will find some good advice and guidelines at the end of the chapter.

Learning from the book

Learning from a book may seem to take longer than learning from a video or teacher, but many people say they remember the sequences better when they read them as they do them. You can make a tape recording of the instructions and play it while you practise. You can also use Dr. Paul Lam's Tai Chi for Arthritis video (*see Resources, page 139*).

Carefully read the instructions and study the images before you attempt the movements. Then progress at your own speed: repeat the movements as often as you need and use the instructions to visualize yourself doing tai chi. Each movement is described in detail. Although tai chi movements flow smoothly from one to the next, the instructions are broken down and described in small segments to make it easier to learn them. As you progress through your practice, the movements will flow together.

Cautions for tai chi practice

This programme is approved for people with arthritis and related conditions by the Arthritis Foundation of Australia. Tai chi, when done slowly and carefully, is safe for most people. However, if your arthritis is particularly severe or painful, please consult your doctor before starting this or any exercise programme.

If there is a medical condition that prevents you from performing the tai chi movements exactly as shown in the following pages, it is quite alright to adapt them to suit your needs. You should always work within your own individual comfort zone, never overstretching yourself and always stopping when you think you are doing too much. Take special care if you've had a knee or hip joint replacement.

If you have any doubts about a posture or a movement, or if you experience discomfort that lasts more than a few hours, please consult your doctor.

Before you begin

Tai chi movements are done slowly and consciously, with your knees slightly bent. Try to focus your mind on each of the movements, and keep your breathing deep and relaxed throughout. You should feel stable, comfortable and balanced as you move your weight from foot to foot through the tai chi steps.

PRACTICAL ADVICE

When you practise tai chi, always work within your own comfort zone and don't try to learn the steps too quickly. Do everything in your own time and at your own pace. The guidelines below will help you to achieve this.

- **Take special care:** move carefully and slowly. If you have a flare (see *page 99*), ask your doctor what exercises are safe for you.
- **Take it slow:** learn one movement at a time. Practise it until you feel confident. Then progress to the next movement. Remember, it is the daily doing of tai chi, not achieving some end goal, that is important.
- **Concentrate:** bring your mind to focus on the movements, which will allow you to be deliberate in what you are doing. Always have a general sense of awareness of what your body is doing.
- **Don't push:** use only the muscles you need. Minimum effort is all that is required for maximum effect. The method will help to relax you and cultivate qi (your vital energy).
- **Be patient:** do not try to do too much too soon. Do not overstretch or overexert yourself. Stay within your comfort range. Progress at a comfortable pace.
- **Be consistent:** practise every day, even if only for a few minutes. Set a regular time to practise. Ten to 20 minutes per day will be sufficient to improve your health and relieve your arthritis. Please check with your doctor or physiotherapist if you are in doubt.

- **Distribute your weight:** if you have difficulty resting most of your weight on one leg, then adjust its distribution so that you are comfortable. You can also straighten your knees if it is uncomfortable to move with bent knees.
- **Know when to stop:** you may feel some mild discomfort at first if you have not been using your muscles regularly. This is normal. But if it feels like pain, stop and rest. As a general guide, if you have pain for more than two hours after you exercise, you may have been overdoing your exercise. You should cut down the length of time or level of exertion, and consult your doctor.

PRECAUTION

When bending your knees, never let the kneecap go beyond the tip of your toes. Your knees may be bent less but not more. If you look down and cannot see your toes, you are bending your knees too much.

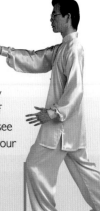

Warming up

Always do these gentle warm-up exercises before you begin tai chi. Remember to do the cooling-down exercises afterwards (*see pages 110–11*). The exercises here have been specially designed for people with arthritis or a related musculoskeletal condition.

Do your warm up and stretching exercises slowly and carefully, progressing at your own pace. Each exercise is done three times, but if that is not comfortable for you, do fewer repetitions. After you've done the warm ups for a few days, you will probably find you feel like doing each three times.

The right stance

Stand in a relaxed but straight posture (*Step 1*). Begin with Ear Drop (*Step 2*) and Head Turns (*Step 3*). These are designed to extend the range of movement in the neck. Next, stretch your spine with Reach the Tree (*overleaf*), keeping your feet flat on the floor if needed for stability.

Lower body

The next three exercises are designed to strengthen and to extend the movement of your lower body. Be sure to have a

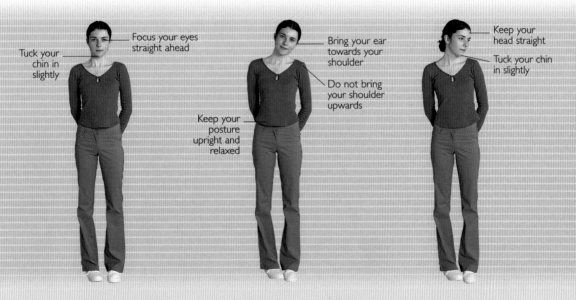

Tuck your chin in slightly

Focus your eyes straight ahead

Keep your posture upright and relaxed

Bring your ear towards your shoulder

Do not bring your shoulder upwards

Keep your head straight

Tuck your chin in slightly

1 Stand upright, relax and imagine your body is aligned on a string passing through your ear, shoulder, hip and heel. Tuck your chin in slightly and focus your eyes straight ahead.

2 Bend your head to the left as far as is comfortable and hold for three seconds. Repeat three times. Bring your head to the centre. Hold for a second. Then repeat the movement, bending your head to the right.

3 Turn your head to look over your left shoulder. Hold for a few seconds. Turn to look over your right shoulder. Hold for a few seconds. Repeat three times. Move on to the next exercise (*overleaf*).

support nearby such as a chair or wall to help you keep your balance.

Kick Back extends the movement in your hips, while Knee Stretch improves the movement of the knees.

If you have trouble with the knee stretch and find it uncomfortable try an alternative. Just stretch out your leg out in front so that your heel touches the ground. Then bring your foot back with your toes touching the ground.

As you gain strength, lift your leg and hold your foot above the ground, increasing the lift a bit more each time you do the exercise.

Guidelines

* Walk around at your own pace for a couple of minutes before you start to do these warm-up movements.
* Move through the exercises slowly and gently, and pay attention to how your body responds.
* Only do as much as is comfortable. Adapt each exercise to your individual situation. If you feel any discomfort or doubt about a particular movement, then don't do it. Consult your doctor or physiotherapist before proceeding.
* At first keep stretches to well within your normal range of motion. You can then

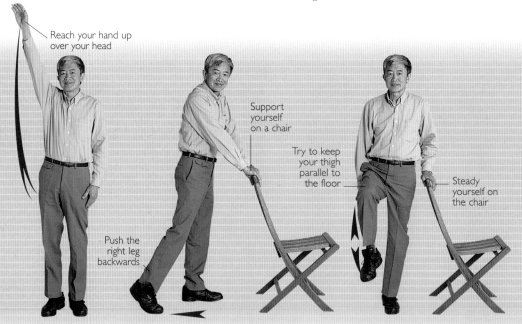

Reach your hand up over your head

Support yourself on a chair

Try to keep your thigh parallel to the floor

Steady yourself on the chair

Push the right leg backwards

REACH THE TREE means standing on your toes and reaching up as though you are picking fruit from a tree. Repeat three times with each hand. Either stand on your toes or keep your feet flat on the ground.

KICK BACK involves standing on the left leg and gently pushing the right leg backwards, within your comfort range, to rest your toes on the ground behind the other foot. Repeat three times and then change legs.

KNEE STRETCH involves standing on one leg and lifting up the other, bending it at the knee. Stretch your lower leg forwards as far as it will comfortably go, and then bend it back. Repeat three times and change legs.

"Always do your warm-up and stretching exercises slowly and carefully."

gradually increase the stretches as your body becomes more flexible.

• One reason for holding a stretch (such as Sideways Stretch) is to allow your muscles to relax. Do not "bounce" as a way of increasing the stretch – bouncing can cause injuries and can actually tighten the muscles you want to loosen.

• Repeat each exercise three times, progress to a maximum of five times, and alternate sides where appropriate.

BENEFITS BOX

The warm-up movements loosen up many of the joints and muscles in your body so that you are ready to take on the more challenging steps in the tai chi programme.

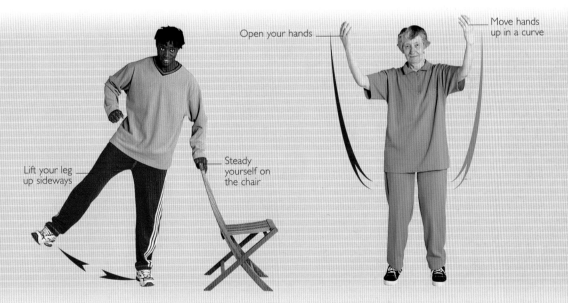

Open your hands

Move hands up in a curve

Lift your leg up sideways

Steady yourself on the chair

SIDEWAYS STRETCH involves standing on your left leg, steadying yourself on a chair and lifting your right leg up sideways. Hold for three seconds and bring it down. Lift only as high as is comfortable and stable. If you can't, don't hold the lift: just raise the leg and then bring it back to the floor. Repeat three times and change legs.

OPEN YOUR HANDS, moving them up in a curve higher than your head as you breathe in. Then bring your arms down in a curve and breathe out. Finish by walking around, clenching and unclenching your hands. Gently move your hands towards your thumb and drop them down gently towards the little fingers.

Cooling down

After completing the tai chi programme, it is important to cool down. Never stop tai chi or any exercise abruptly: take the time to allow your body to return to a resting level and to settle your energy.

It may not seem as though you have been moving around much, but actually you will have done quite a bit of work with your knees and arms. So it is mportant to take a few minutes to loosen your body and wind down. You will also want to perform an exercise to conserve the *qi* you have generated.

An alternative to the cool–down exercises illustrated here is to repeat the warming–up exercises (*see pages 107–9*).

Shake out your legs

Shift your weight to your left foot. Bend your right knee back, and "kick" your right foot forwards, allowing it to come back to the ground. Shift your weight to your right foot, and then bend your left knee back and "kick" your left foot forwards, allowing it to return to the ground. These are not big kicks: your foot should just swing easily

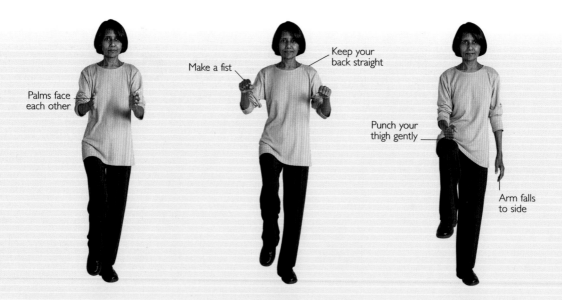

Palms face each other

Make a fist

Keep your back straight

Punch your thigh gently

Arm falls to side

1 Stand upright and relax. Bring both your hands out in front of you and raise your right knee up as far as is comfortable for you. Keep your left foot firmly on the floor.

2 Keeping your back straight, form a loose fist with both your hands and raise your right knee a little higher if you can. Be sure to move only as far as is comfortable for you.

3 If you can, raise the knee a little higher and gently punch your right thigh with your right fist, and let your left arm fall to the side. Repeat three times and change legs.

"Never finish your tai chi exercises abruptly – you need to relax slowly."

forwards, as you allow your leg to relax. Repeat three times for each leg.

If this is uncomfortable, just stretch each leg out in front so that only your heel touches the ground. Then bring your foot back with your toes touching the ground.

After doing the exercises below, it is a good idea to walk around clenching and unclenching your hands by making and relaxing fists. Then give your feet and hands a few gentle shakes.

BENEFITS BOX

The cooling-down movements enable the joints and muscles of your body to return to a state of relaxation. They also conserve the qi you have generated during your tai chi exercises.

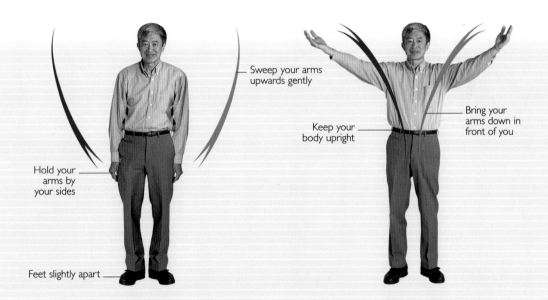

Sweep your arms upwards gently

Keep your body upright

Bring your arms down in front of you

Hold your arms by your sides

Feet slightly apart

1 Stand with your feet slightly apart at a distance comfortable for you. Let your arms hang by your sides and gently open your palms. Raise both your arms together and move them up in a curve higher than your head and breathe in.

2 Keep your body upright but relaxed and keep your chin tucked in slightly. Lower your arms and, as you do so, press the palms of your hands down gently in a curve in front of you and breathe out. Repeat this three times.

Tai chi walking

Before you begin the programme, it will help to learn the tai chi style of walking forwards and backwards (*see below*), and sideways (*see page113*). The idea behind these exercise sequences is to give you a basic foundation, making it easier to learn the Tai Chi for Arthritis programme.

Follow the sequence below and repeat it several times at your own speed. Then, do the same walk in reverse, lifting the left foot first. Always be sure the distance between your feet is comfortable for you and that you feel balanced.

To walk sideways, repeat the sequence of Steps 1 to 4 on page 113 several times until you are confident and then do the same walk in reverse, lifting the left foot first.

General rules:
* When you walk forwards, make sure the heel touches down first.
* When moving backwards, make sure the ball of the foot touches down first.
* When moving sideways, move your feet parallel to each other. The ball of the foot touches down first, then the whole foot.

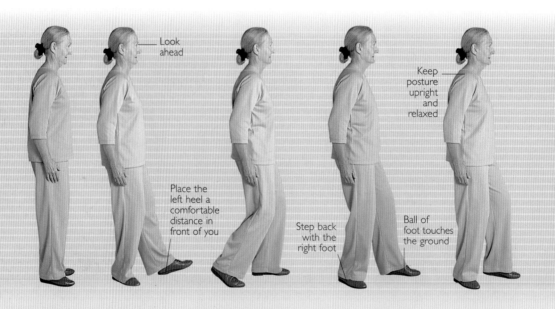

Look ahead

Keep posture upright and relaxed

Place the left heel a comfortable distance in front of you

Step back with the right foot

Ball of foot touches the ground

WALKING FORWARDS AND BACKWARDS

Start in the standing position with your heels close together and your toes pointing out-wards. Bend your knees slightly, lift up your left foot and step forwards with the left heel.

As you transfer your weight forwards onto the left foot, lift up the right leg and place the ball of the foot near the left heel. To reverse the sequence, step backwards with the right

foot, letting the ball touch the ground first, followed by the whole foot. As you transfer your weight back onto your right foot, lift up the left foot and bring it slightly backwards.

THE STANDING POSITION

Stand comfortably with your heels close to each other and toes pointing outward at about 90 degrees. Check your posture: you should be upright but relaxed.

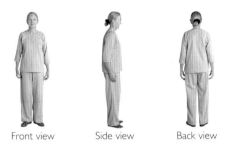

Front view   Side view   Back view

"Feel a relaxed connection between the feet, lower back, waist and arms."

BENEFITS BOX

Tai chi walking trains you to consciously centre your weight on one leg, then step out with the other. When you're ready you transfer your weight onto the other leg. This improves your balance and gait.

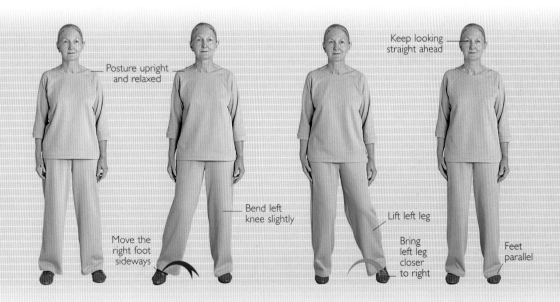

Posture upright and relaxed

Move the right foot sideways

Bend left knee slightly

Keep looking straight ahead

Lift left leg

Bring left leg closer to right

Feet parallel

1 Stand with both feet approximately shoulder–width apart and parallel to each other. Check your posture: you should be upright but relaxed.

2 Move your weight onto the left foot, bending the left knee slightly. Lift and move the right foot sideways comfortably, with the ball touching first.

3 As you transfer your weight back to your right foot, lift the left foot until only the ball is touching the ground and bring it closer to the right.

4 Return to the same position as Step 1, with your feet half to one shoulders' width apart and parallel. Your posture is upright but relaxed.

MOVEMENT ONE

Beginning

The opening movements of the programme are also called the Commencement Form. Your starting posture should be upright and relaxed, not rigid. To align your body, recall the first posture of the warm–up routine (*see page 107*) and imagine a straight line drawn down through your ear to your shoulder, hip and heel. Now imagine a string going up from the crown of your head, gently pulling you upright.

Next, cleanse your mind of daily cares: take a deep breath in and, as you breathe out, empty your mind of all thoughts and let your worries flow away. Bring all your concentration to the movements you are about to do and try to hold that focus throughout your tai chi practice.

The overall sequence of this Beginning movement is as follows: slowly bring your hands up in front of you as you breathe in, then bring your hands down slowly as you breathe out. Take a step forwards with your left foot, and as your right foot follows to join it, push your hands forwards.

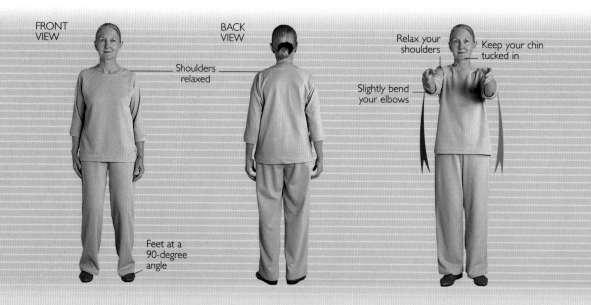

FRONT VIEW

BACK VIEW

Shoulders relaxed

Feet at a 90-degree angle

Relax your shoulders

Keep your chin tucked in

Slightly bend your elbows

1 Stand with your heels almost touching and your feet forming a 90–degree angle. If this is not comfortable for you, move your feet a bit further apart. Look straight ahead and tuck your chin in slightly. Relax your knees and shoulders and let your arms hang by your sides.

2 Breathe in, bringing your arms slowly up and out in front of you to approximately shoulder height. Keep the palms of your hands facing each other and separated by a shoulder's width.

SIDE VIEW

It is important to keep your body upright with your back straight, neither leaning backwards or forwards. Keep your knees slightly bent and relax into your hips.

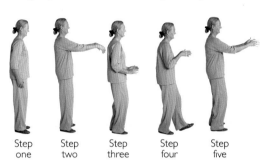

| Step one | Step two | Step three | Step four | Step five |

"Empty your mind of all thoughts and let your worries flow away."

BENEFITS BOX

Cleansing your mind and focusing on your body as it moves will help you to switch off from a stressful situation and achieve tranquillity of mind more easily.

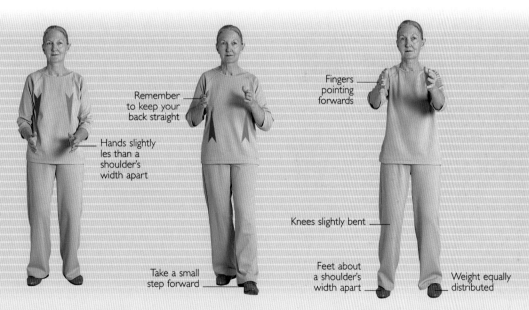

Remember to keep your back straight

Hands slightly les than a shoulder's width apart

Fingers pointing forwards

Knees slightly bent

Take a small step forward

Feet about a shoulder's width apart

Weight equally distributed

3 Now breathe out, bringing your arms down slowly to hip level and, at the same time, bending your knees slightly. Your hands end up in front of your hips with the palms facing each other.

4 Bring your arms up to chest height. Shift your weight onto your right foot. Step your left foot forwards, keeping the knee straight but not stiff and making sure that the heel touches the ground first.

5 Shift your weight forwards onto your left foot, allowing your knee to bend. At the same time, push your hands forwards as if passing a ball to someone. Bring your right foot up in line with your left.

MOVEMENT TWO

Opening & Closing Hands

Following on from the last step of the Beginning sequence, Opening & Closing Hands is one of the simple but powerful qigong movements that are a feature of Sun style tai chi.

It is helpful to imagine that, between your hands, a gentle magnetic field creates a resistance against which you must work. In Step 2 you have to pull slowly but gently against this force. In Step 3 you have to push against it to bring your hands towards each other.

The overall sequence of this movement is as follows: bring your hands in towards you, open your hands and breathe in, then finally close your hands and breathe out.

BENEFITS BOX

Breathing slowly and deeply with the aid of upper body movement improves lung capacity and the flow of qi. Strong qi will make you healthier and more relaxed.

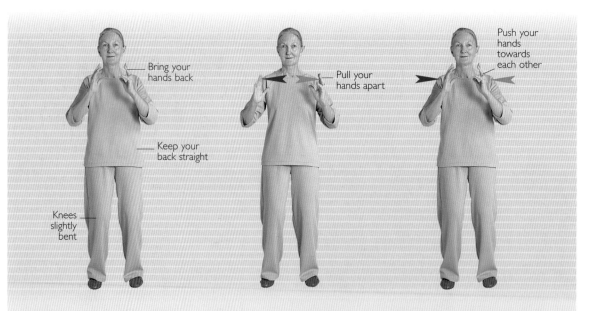

Bring your hands back

Keep your back straight

Knees slightly bent

Pull your hands apart

Push your hands towards each other

1 Bring your hands in front of your chest at a distance comfortable for you. Your hands are separated by the width of your head and your palms face each other with the fingers pointing upwards.

2 Breathe in and, as you do so, open up your hands slowly to approximately a shoulder's width. If your knees are tired now, you can slowly straighten up as your separate your hands.

3 As you breathe out, gently push your hands towards one another. If you straightened your knees in the last step, you can now bend them slowly as you move your hands towards each other.

MOVEMENT THREE
Single Whip

This graceful and classic tai chi movement follows on from the last step of Opening & Closing Hands.

In Step 1 you should be careful to step to the right at a distance comfortable for you. This will probably be somewhere between one and two feet (30–50cm). Remember, do not step too far at first.

The overall sequence is: turn towards your right, step out with your right foot, open hands out wide while, following the left hand with your gaze.

"Put your hands against an invisible wall and gaze over your left hand."

BENEFITS BOX

You will learn to transfer your weight in a controlled manner, maintaining an upright and relaxed posture. This improves muscular strength, balance and coordination.

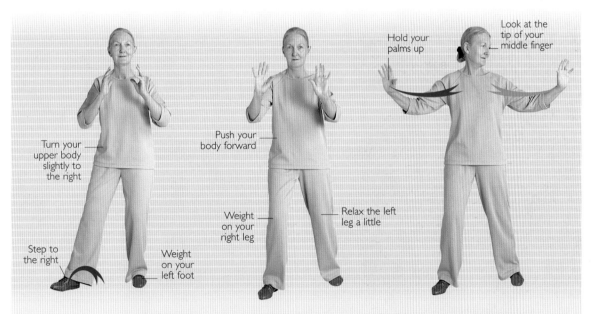

Turn your upper body slightly to the right

Step to the right

Weight on your left foot

Push your body forward

Weight on your right leg

Hold your palms up

Look at the tip of your middle finger

Relax the left leg a little

1 Turn your upper body slightly to the right, moving from your hip. Shift your weight to your left foot and step your right foot to the right and slightly forwards. Let the heel touch the ground first.

2 Shift your weight gradually onto your right leg and push your hands forwards, turning your hands so that both palms are facing towards the front. Let your left knee relax a little.

3 Turn your upper body very slightly to the left and extend your arms to the sides. Both hands are parallel and roughly symmetrical. Hold your hands as if putting your palms up against an invisible wall.

MOVEMENT FOUR

Waving Hands in the Clouds

This tai chi sequence, which follows on from the last step of the Single Whip, consists of three parts. The second and third part are exact repetitions of the first. Together they generate energy.

In the illustrated steps below, the first part begins with Step 1 and ends with Step 4. Practise these first until you are confident with the overall movement.

To help you with the link between the first two parts, the second part begins with Step 5 (the same as Step 1) and then

Step 6 (the same as Step 2). The third part repeats the second part.

We recommend that you practise the first part several times because it is quite a difficult movement. When you are confident enough you can continue with the second and third. Then you can practise all three together as a single, continuous movement.

When you attempt all three parts of the complete sequence, remember that you will be taking three steps to the

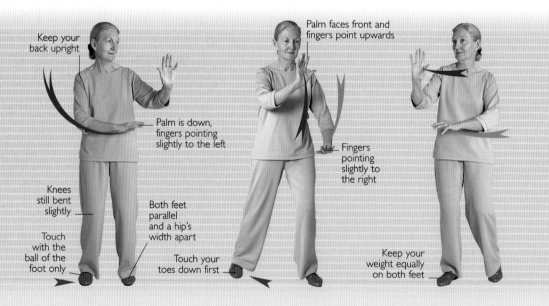

Keep your back upright

Palm is down, fingers pointing slightly to the left

Knees still bent slightly

Touch with the ball of the foot only

Both feet parallel and a hip's width apart

Touch your toes down first

Palm faces front and fingers point upwards

Fingers pointing slightly to the right

Keep your weight equally on both feet

1 Transfer your weight onto your left foot and bring the right hand down in a gentle curve near to your left elbow. At the same time, bring your right foot to your left, with most of your weight on your left foot.

2 Bring your left hand down ending with palm facing the ground. Lift your right hand up in a curve to shoulder height. At the same time, step your right foot comfortably to the right, keeping it in line with your left.

3 Gradually transfer your weight to the right foot. Move your upper body and arms to the right, bringing your left foot in line with your right so your feet are about half a shoulder's width apart.

"Feel the rhythmic movement of your body as you transfer your weight."

right – so you will need to allow yourself plenty of space in the room where you practise your tai chi.

One feature is the rhythmic movement of your body as you transfer your weight from one foot to another as you make the three graceful steps to your right.

The three parts effectively consist of 12 steps. The sequence ends on the final, or 13th step, when you turn your upper body and arms to the left.

BENEFITS BOX

Your upper arms form an energy field to enhance your qi. Stepping sideways improves lower limb strength. The rhythmic transferring of weight gently exercises the knee joints, improving flexibility.

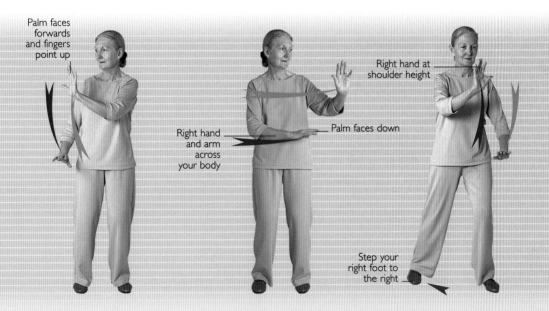

Palm faces forwards and fingers point up

Right hand and arm across your body

Right hand at shoulder height

Palm faces down

Step your right foot to the right

4 Bring your left hand up to shoulder height towards your right arm. At the same time, bring the right hand down to hip level with palm facing the ground and fingers pointing slightly to the left.

5 Turn your upper body and arms to the left as you shift your weight to your left foot. Your right hand and arm move across your your body with the palm down and fingers slightly pointing left.

6 Bring your left hand down ending with palm facing down. Lift the right hand up in a curve to shoulder height. At the same time, step your right foot comfortably to the right, keeping it in line with your left.

MOVEMENT FIVE

Opening & Closing Hands

This is a repeat of the Opening & Closing Hands sequence on page 116. This time it follows on from the final step of Waving Hands in the Clouds where the upper body and hands were facing left.

As before it is helpful to imagine that, between your hands, a gentle magnetic field creates a resistance against which you must work. In Step 2 you have to pull slowly but gently against this force. In Step 3 you have to push against it to bring your hands towards each other.

The overall sequence of this movement is: bring your hands in, then open your hands and breathe in, then close hands and breathe out.

You can use mental imagery and visualization to direct your breath into your abdomen. This will have the beneficial effect of opening up more air space in your lungs and improving the flow of *qi* in your system. Stronger *qi* contributes to better health and helps to relieve pain and stress.

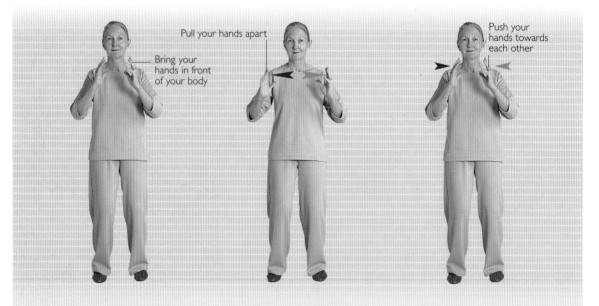

Pull your hands apart

Bring your hands in front of your body

Push your hands towards each other

1 Bring your hands in front of your chest, with palms facing each other and fingers pointing upwards. Your knees are still slightly bent, your back is straight and your weight is equally on both feet.

2 Breathe in and, as you do so, open up your hands slowly to approximately a shoulder's width apart. If your knees have become tired, you can slowly stand up straight as you separate your hands.

3 As you breathe out, gently push your hands towards one another. If you straightened up during the previous step, you can now bend your knees slowly as you bring your hands closer together.

MOVEMENT SIX

Closing Movement

All through the six Basic Movements you have been gathering *qi* within you as well as stimulating its flow in your body, and now you need to let it settle.

With this Closing Movement you are returning to a posture similar but not the same as Step 1 of Beginning (*see page 114*). The difference is that here your feet are parallel and not at a 90-degree angle.

Make sure you are confident with the Basic Movements before moving on to learn the six Advanced Movements.

"Allow the qi you have gathered within you time to settle."

BENEFITS BOX

Slowly stopping your movement and standing still for a little while allows your qi to settle. It trains you to build the good habit of finishing your daily task properly and to avoid rushing unnecessarily.

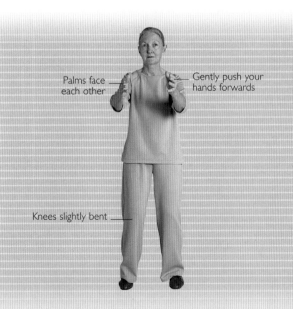

Palms face each other — Gently push your hands forwards

Knees slightly bent —

1 Stretch your hands out gently in front of you at approximately shoulder height, with the fingers pointing forwards and palms facing each other. Your hands should be separated by a shoulder's width and your knees should be slightly bent.

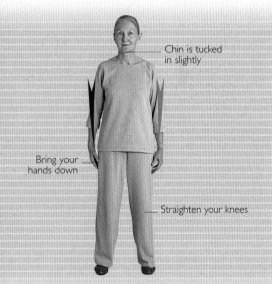

Chin is tucked in slightly

Bring your hands down —

— Straighten your knees

2 Bring your hands down slowly to the side of your thighs and, at the same time, slowly straighten your knees and stand upright. Tuck your chin in and relax your knees and shoulders. Make sure your posture is upright and your back straight.

The Six Advanced Movements

The following series of advanced tai chi movements is more challenging than the Basic Movements. But don't hurry to start learning them until you feel confident and comfortable enough to progress; and don't push yourself beyond your limits.

Reaching a more "advanced" level in tai chi is not essential or important. Try to remember that it is the process of learning and practising tai chi – and not the effort you put in nor the level of expertise you attain – that will improve your overall health and will help you to cope with your arthritis symptoms.

Putting the movements together

Before you begin this advanced series, it is important for you to have a foundation in tai chi. You should have learned and regularly practised the six Basic Movements for at least three weeks. The six Advanced Movements join directly to the six Basic Movements: Brush Knee, the first movement of the advanced series, follows on from Opening & Closing Hands, the fifth movement of the Basic series.

Together, these two series provide you with a complete sequence of 12 movements – the first five of the Basic, the six advanced and the final Closing Movement. Eventually, you will learn to perform this sequence in one graceful flowing choreography of movement. The whole sequence will provide you with a short tai chi form that, practised regularly every day, can help to bring you improved health and greater well-being.

Finally, at the end of this chapter, you will find a set of basic qigong exercises that will help to relax you. At the same time, they will enhance precious *qi* energy in your system that will invigorate your body, mind and spirit. You can practise the qigong exercises either as a separate sequence or after the 12 tai chi movements.

Taking tai chi further

Once you have mastered the 12 movements and feel confident you can perform them with ease, you may want to study tai chi in more depth. The best way would be to find a tai chi teacher who suits your needs. You will find some guidelines on what to look out for at the end of the chapter.

At home, the most important way to advance your tai chi and improve your health is to practise regularly every day. This practice can take as little as ten minutes, or as long as you like: it is the regular practice that is important, not how long you do it.

By practising with total concentration, you can gain deeper experience of the principles of tai chi and a more profound sense of union with your mind, body and spirit. To help develop the meditative aspects of tai chi, read more about qigong and the essential principles of tai chi (*see Resources, page 140*).

To develop internal force as well as strength, imagine, whenever you do tai chi, that the air is dense and seems to resist you – and you have to gently push it.

Finally, learn to do some of the movements, or even the whole set, in reverse. This adds variety to your exercise, will make the sequence longer and give better balance between left and right sides.

QIGONG EXERCISES
The breathing, movement and meditation techniques of qigong enhance *qi* energy and bring power and strength to your tai chi practice.

MOVEMENT ONE

Brush Knee

This opening movement follows on from the third step of Opening & Closing Hands (*see page 120*). In this posture you gently brought your hands together in front of your chest, while breathing out.

In Step 2 of Brush Knee you will step your left foot to the left – if you find this difficult or uncomfortable then make it easier by turning your right foot slightly inwards first.

To execute the Brush Knee movement properly you need to focus your mental concentration on the coordination of your whole body. The benefits come through achieving controlled motion, which will in time improve your muscular strength, flexibility and coordination.

The overall sequence of this movement is: turn slightly to the right, stretching out your right hand; then step to the left and, as you brush your left hand past your left knee, turn to the left and push your right hand forwards as if you are pushing someone's chest away.

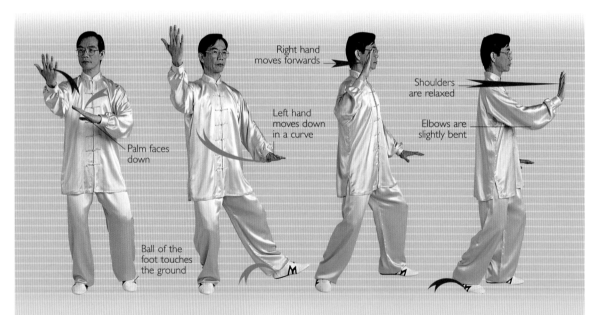

Right hand moves forwards

Left hand moves down in a curve

Palm faces down

Ball of the foot touches the ground

Shoulders are relaxed

Elbows are slightly bent

1 Turn right, extend the right arm and bring the left near the right elbow. Shift your weight to the right foot while you lift the left foot towards it.

2 Step your left foot to the left with your heel touching the ground. Extend your right hand further and move the left down in a curve to your hip.

3 Turn towards the left. Brush the left hand past the left knee and bring the right hand up near your right ear as if pushing forwards.

4 Continue to push your right hand and, at the same time, step your right foot behind your left foot, with only the ball touching the ground.

MOVEMENT TWO

Playing the Lute

This movement, which continues on from Brush Knee, looks as though you are playing the strings of a lute. In Step 2 push your hands smoothly past one another. As you do so, imagine a pole with a diameter of about 10cm (4ins) between them and your palms moving along its surface.

In Step 3, the half step the left foot takes is known as an "empty step". Almost all your weight is on one leg while the foot of the other just touches the ground.

"Feel the energy as you brush your hands past each other."

BENEFITS BOX

The subtle transfer of your weight in this movement trains you to be aware of, and to control, even minor shifts in body weight. This will help to prevent a fall and to improve your gait.

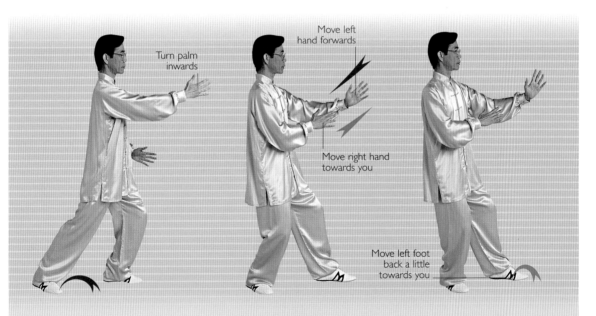

Turn palm inwards

Move left hand forwards

Move right hand towards you

Move left foot back a little towards you

1 Step your right foot back half a step and stretch your right hand forwards, turning your palm inwards. Turn the left palm inwards so it is facing right. The toes of your feet will form a 45–degree angle.

2 Gradually transfer more of your weight onto your right foot. At the same time, move your left hand up and pull your right arm towards you. It is as if the hands are sliding past each other.

3 Continue moving your arms until the right hand is near the left elbow and the left hand extends at eye level. At the same time, bring the left foot back a little, with the ball touching the ground.

MOVEMENT THREE

Parry & Punch

This long, challenging sequence involves a blend of steps, transfer of weight, movement of both hands, as well as making a fist. All in all, you will take three and a half steps so make sure you have plenty of room in which to move.

One notable feature of the sequence is the way the force of your body moving forwards onto the front foot gives a momentum to the push or punch of the hands.

In Step 2, your hands will push smoothly past each other in a similar but reverse step to Playing the Lute (*see page 125*). So you can use the same analogy of moving your hands smoothly along a pole about 10cm (4ins) in diameter. On a couple of occasions in this sequence – for example, in Step 3 – you will take a step forwards that

MAKING A FIST
The fist should be loose and comfortable, with the thumb bent over the middle of the index and middle fingers.

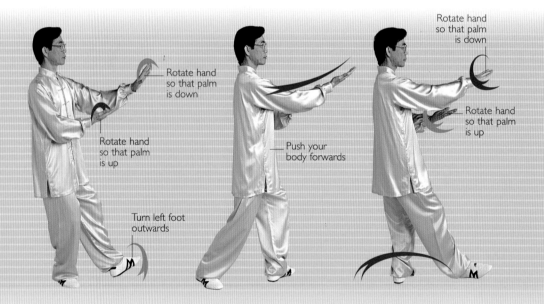

Rotate hand so that palm is down

Rotate hand so that palm is up

Turn left foot outwards

Push your body forwards

Rotate hand so that palm is down

Rotate hand so that palm is up

1 Lift your left foot slightly, turning the toes outwards and placing your left heel on the ground. At the same time, rotate your hands so that your left palm is down and your right palm is up.

2 As you transfer your weight forwards onto your left foot, use the force and momentum of your body to push your right hand forwards. At the same time, pull the left hand back towards you.

3 Turn both hands as you step the right foot forwards, placing the heel on the ground first. Your toes will be pointing slightly to the right. Your left palm is facing down and your right palm is facing up.

"Transmit the momentum from your moving body into the push and punch."

you may find a little uncomfortable. Do not try to force the step. Instead, make sure you place your foot in a position that is stable and comfortable for you. As with many tai chi steps, the movements will become easier the more you practise.

In Step 5, you are asked to turn your left palm down before making a fist. This is like a martial art move designed to block a punch that someone might be throwing at you.

BENEFITS BOX

Tai chi movements are slow, even and continuous. To control the flow and rhythm of movement helps improve posture, body awareness and muscle strength. This long sequence benefits mobility and memory.

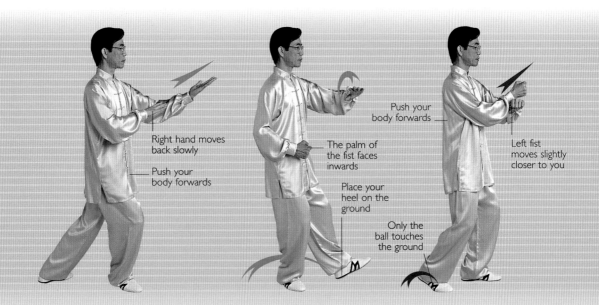

Right hand moves back slowly

Push your body forwards

Push your body forwards

The palm of the fist faces inwards

Place your heel on the ground

Left fist moves slightly closer to you

Only the ball touches the ground

4 As you transfer your weight forwards onto your right foot, use the momentum and force of your body to push your left hand forwards. At the same time, pull the right hand back towards you.

5 Turn your left palm down and make a fist. Bend your elbow to bring it closer to your body. At the same time, bring the right hand down near your hip, making a fist. Step your left foot forwards.

6 As you transfer your weight forwards onto your left foot, bring your left fist slightly closer to you. As you take half a step forwards with your right foot, push your right fist forwards just above the left wrist.

MOVEMENT FOUR

Block & Close

In this short sequence you are gathering energy as a prelude to making the push in the next movement, Embracing the Tiger, Pushing the Mountain.

The stepping back movement in Block & Close is not one that is often done normally Yet you might need to do this suddenly during an accident, which could lead to a loss of balance. Consequently, this exercise helps to develop the muscles for moving backwards, so minimizing your chance of injury.

At the end of Step 2, your left foot makes a slight move backwards towards the right foot. This is another "empty step", similar to the one in Step 5 of Playing the Lute (*see page 125*).

Almost all of your weight is rested on your right foot and the right side of your body. Meanwhile, the ball of your left foot is barely touching the ground. It is as if your left leg is poised, free of your weight and ready to move forwards when it is necessary.

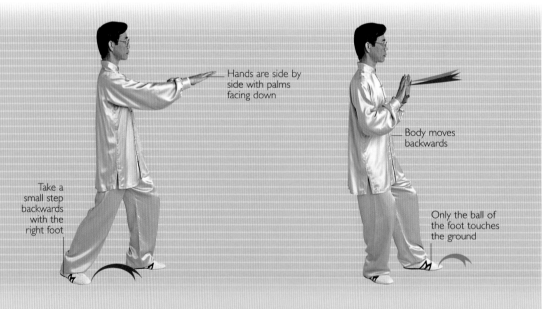

Hands are side by side with palms facing down

Take a small step backwards with the right foot

Body moves backwards

Only the ball of the foot touches the ground

1 Open up both hands and separate them. Stretch them out in front of you with the palms facing down and take a small step backwards with the right foot, touching the ground only with the ball of the foot.

2 As you move your weight onto the right foot, bring both hands back in a gentle curve in front of your chest. Bring your left foot back slightly, with only the ball of the foot touching the ground. This is an "empty step".

MOVEMENT FIVE

Embracing the Tiger, Pushing the Mountain

This poetically named movement is important for mobilizing the *qi* energy flow within you and so has beneficial healing effects. During the movement you will be mentally focused so that you can push gently and effectively with your inner strength.

Step 1 is Embracing the Tiger when you gather up within you the energy and power necessary to Push the Mountain in Step 2. The force of the push comes from the body's forward movement as you transfer your weight onto the left foot. Imagine there is a resistance coming to meet your pushing hands.

BENEFITS BOX

The rhythmic movement will open up qi channels and improve qi circulation. The qi propels blood and body fluid and so enhances healing and vitality.

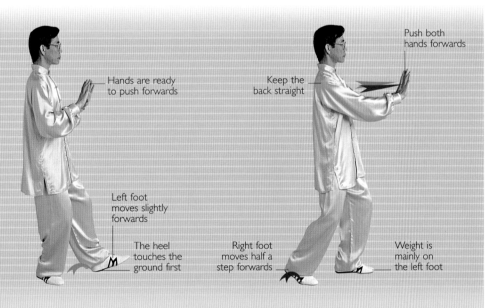

Hands are ready to push forwards

Keep the back straight

Push both hands forwards

Left foot moves slightly forwards

The heel touches the ground first

Right foot moves half a step forwards

Weight is mainly on the left foot

1 Take a small step forwards with your left foot, with your heel touching the ground first. Imagine you are stepping slightly forwards and, at the same time, pushing your opponent away. That is why it is called Pushing the Mountain.

2 Transfer your weight forwards onto your left foot. Push both hands forwards as you take half a step forwards with the right foot, touching the ground with the toes. The right foot will be about 10cm (4ins) behind the left foot.

MOVEMENT SIX

Opening & Closing Hands

The last part of the series of six Advanced Movements, Opening & Closing Hands is the same powerful qigong exercise you learned in the second and fifth movement of the basic series.

The simple steps will enhance your *qi*, improving its circulation and calming the mind and body, which helps relieve stress and depression.

As before, try to imagine that, between your hands, there is a gentle magnetic field creating a resistance against which you must move your hands. In Step 2 you have to pull slowly and gently against the force. In Step 3 you have to push against it in order to bring your hands towards each other.

The overall sequence of this movement is as follows: bring your hands in, open your hands and breathe in, then finally close your hands and breathe out.

In Step 2 you may find your knees become tired. If so, you can slowly stand up straight as you separate your hands.

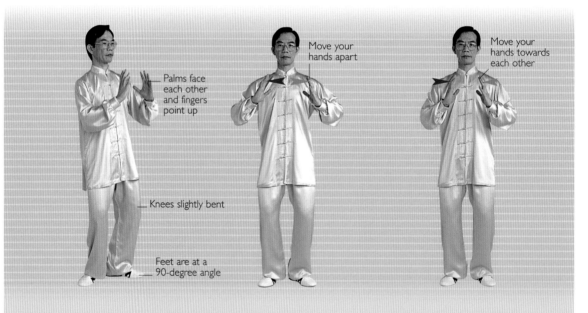

Palms face each other and fingers point up

Knees slightly bent

Feet are at a 90-degree angle

Move your hands apart

Move your hands towards each other

1 Move the heel of your right foot inwards to the left heel at a distance comfortable for you. Lift and turn your left foot slightly inwards and bring your hands in front of your chest.

2 As you breathe in open up your hands slowly to about a shoulder's width apart. If your knees have become tired, then slowly straighten them as you separate your hands.

3 As you breathe out, gently push your hands towards one another. If you straightened up in the previous step, bend your knees slowly as you bring your hands closer together.

MOVEMENT SEVEN
Closing Movement

The purpose of this Closing Movement is to relax and focus your concentration so that you can slowly return to where you started. You have now come full circle and returned to the first position at the beginning of the 12-movement set.

This has a significance reminiscent of the *yin–yang* symbol (*see page 80*) used to represent tai chi. As in nature, the circle has no beginning or end. The beginning point leads us back to the end point, which is the same as the beginning.

"Return your whole body to its original position in an orderly fashion."

BENEFITS BOX

*This movement restores the qi back to its storage house in the **dan tian** (three fingers' breadth below the navel) and so establishes tranquillity.*

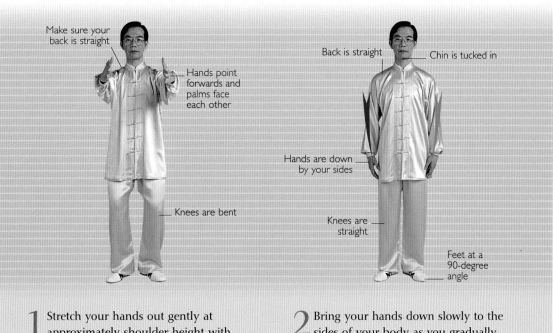

Make sure your back is straight

Hands point forwards and palms face each other

Knees are bent

Back is straight

Chin is tucked in

Hands are down by your sides

Knees are straight

Feet at a 90-degree angle

1 Stretch your hands out gently at approximately shoulder height with your fingers pointing forwards and your palms facing each other. Your hands will be separated by about a shoulder's width and your knees slightly bent.

2 Bring your hands down slowly to the sides of your body as you gradually straighten your knees and stand upright. Return your whole body to its original posture – upright and relaxed, chin tucked in and heels touching.

Qigong sequence

Qigong is a Chinese system of internal energy exercises designed to stimulate the flow of blood flow and to improve the circulation of *qi*. It builds up strength and stamina, and clears the mind and body of unwanted blockages of energy.

One word of warning: qigong exercises can be deceptively powerful and so it is important that you do not practise the sequence of movements illustrated here if you are over-tired, emotionally upset, ill or have just eaten heavily.

Preparing to do qigong

Choose a quiet place where you will not be disturbed for 10 or 15 minutes. Many people prefer to be outdoors for their qigong practice – the place should not be too hot, windy or wet. If you practise inside then make sure the room is well–ventilated.

Wear loose-fitting clothes if you can but if not then make sure you remove anything that is constricting, such as watch or belt.

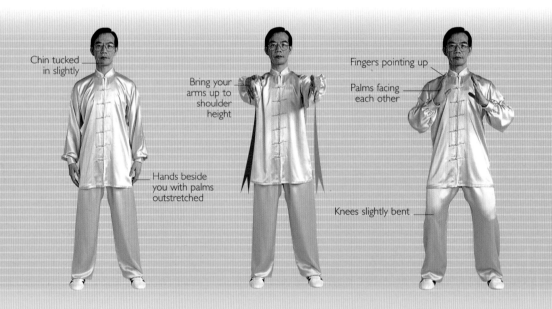

Chin tucked in slightly

Bring your arms up to shoulder height

Fingers pointing up

Palms facing each other

Hands beside you with palms outstretched

Knees slightly bent

1 Stand upright and relaxed with your eyes looking straight ahead and your feet a shoulder's width apart. Tuck your chin in slightly and relax your shoulders with your arms by your sides.

2 As you breathe in, bring your arms up slowly to shoulder height so they are straight in front of you. Keep your palms facing each other. Your elbows should be slightly bent and shoulders relaxed.

3 As you breathe out, bring your arms slowly in to within 10cm (4ins) of your chest and bend your knees slightly. Your palms should be facing each other with fingers pointing upwards.

"Feel the relaxed connection between the feet, lower back, waist and arms."

Before beginning qigong be sure to warm up (*see pages 107–9*) and afterwards do the cooling–down exercises (*see pages 110–11*).

You can repeat this qigong sequence as many times as you like so long as you are comfortable and not pushing yourself too hard. A good regime is to complete the sequence three times for the first three weeks, increasing this gradually over several weeks to six and then nine times at each session. (*Continued overleaf.*)

BENEFITS BOX

Qigong improves posture, increases stamina and develops inner power without putting a physical strain on the body. It strengthens the immune system and so helps to combat illness.

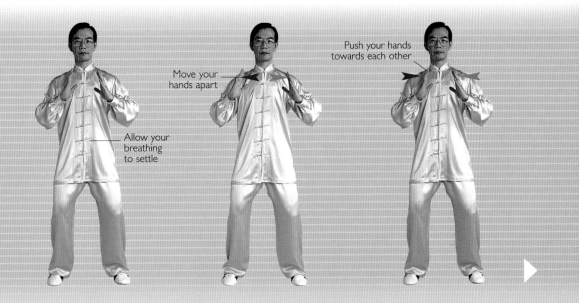

Move your hands apart

Push your hands towards each other

Allow your breathing to settle

4 Maintain this posture while you allow your body and breathing to settle. Your mind should be focused and calm, your body upright but relaxed, with your chin tucked slightly in and knees slightly bent.

5 As you breathe in, slowly pull your hands apart to a shoulder's width. Imagine pulling slowly against a gentle magnetic field that attracts your palms and prevents you from opening your hands.

6 As you breathe out, gently push your hands together, but don't let them touch. Imagine you can feel a slight resistance, as though the force is now working in reverse. Move on to Step 7 (*overleaf*).

Your body

When you stand in the starting position make sure your body is upright and relaxed, but not rigid. Take your time to let your breathing settle. Imagine you are aligned as though a string were passing through your ear, shoulder, hip and heel, and pulling gently up through the top of your head.

Tuck your chin in slightly. Unlock your knees and elbows, and use only as much effort as it takes to keep you standing upright, with no extra tension.

Your breathing

Become aware of your breath flowing in and out. Breathe slowly and easily, thinking of your breathing as the tide coming in and out, without any effort, as though "it were breathing you". Allow your in-breaths and out-breaths to coordinate with your movements.

As you breathe through your nose, imagine the air travelling through your airways to your lungs and then down to your abdomen. Allow your abdomen to expand slightly as you breathe in, and

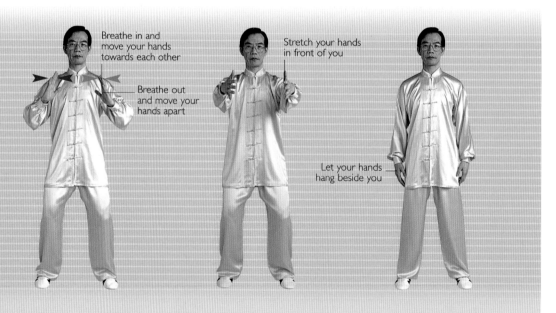

Breathe in and move your hands towards each other

Breathe out and move your hands apart

Stretch your hands in front of you

Let your hands hang beside you

7 Repeat the opening and closing movements (*Steps 5 and 6*) three times. Perform the movements slowly and smoothly, and coordinate them with your breathing.

8 To finish the qigong exercise: at the completion of a hand closing movement, stretch your hands out in front of you as though you were about to hand a ball to someone.

9 Bring your elbows in towards you, letting your arms straighten. Bring them to rest at your sides as you straighten your legs slowly and breathe out.

then to contract as you breathe out. Let your tongue gently touch your upper palate. As the air travels out imagine it coming up from your abdomen to your lungs, through your airways and finally out through your nose. This is called diaphragmatic, or abdominal, breathing (*see pages 92–93*).

Your mind

Before you begin your qigong practice, cleanse and focus your mind. Allow yourself to settle into your breathing. Let any worries or thoughts flow away on each out–breath. Think of something peaceful and serene. Visualize yourself in a place that is safe and calming for you. Many people imagine they are outside, perhaps in a deep and silent forest, or alone on a beach at sunset.

In Step 7, focus your mind on the simple opening and closing actions, so that you are concentrated on the action.

If your mind begins to wander, bring it back to focus on the movement. If your concentration continues to wander, visualize a tranquil and serene place, or simply focus on your breathing. If you are still unable to concentrate, stop and try again later.

When you visualize the magnetic force in the opening and closing movements (*see Steps 5 and 6*), you can feel the *qi* grow between your hands. You can then imagine *qi* flowing through your body, easing stiffness and pain, and bringing light and energy to each tender place.

RETAINING YOUR QI

During the qigong sequence, you have cultivated some precious qi energy which needs to be retained to benefit your body and spirit. An exercise called "washing" your qi – it is like the motions you might make when massaging – does just that. It also gives your body a gentle and relaxing massage.

- Do the exercise slowly and carefully, keeping your body relaxed.
- Stand with your hands at your sides. Stretch your arms out to the sides with your palms up and slowly raise your arms up above your head. Bring your hands to rest on the top of your head.
- Now draw your hands around, over and down both sides of your body, making a complete circuit.
- Gently draw your hands back over the top of your head, down your neck and around your neck to your shoulders and chest.
- Continue slowly and steadily, moving your hands down your ribcage and then around to the back of your chest, down your waist and buttocks, and down the outside of the legs, bending down to draw your hands around to the front of your toes. Bend only as far as is comfortable.
- Now bring your hands up the inside of your thighs and the front of your chest to your face and then over your head as you go back down again. Don't touch your toes if you cannot reach them comfortably.
- Repeat this three times. Come to rest standing comfortably with your hands by your side. Feel yourself relaxed and at the centre of your body, mind and spirit.
- You have completed your qigong exercise.

Finding a tai chi teacher

Many people will be happy to continue practising the tai chi movements they have learned in this book, gaining the benefits daily and feeling the symptoms of their arthritis ease.

Others will want to build on their experience and explore new steps and new forms. There are increasing numbers of people learning tai chi and its popularity means there are more and more teachers.

Finding the right teacher for you can present problems – there may not be a good class in your neighbourhood or the teacher may be asking you to do things that don't seem to be right. Look for the good qualities (*see right*) in a tai chi teacher and for some of the danger signs (*see box, page 137*), and decide for yourself the kind of teacher you need.

Moving on to other styles

Don't be in a rush to move on and learn more "complicated" or "harder" styles of tai chi. You can progress in your skill and level of tai chi within the 12 movements in this book. The simple forms, done regularly, have great benefit even for those who are advanced practitioners of tai chi. Also, some people may prefer not to memorize many more movements. Students and instructors should continue to practise these basic sets for a considerable time.

However, some people may prefer to learn more variations or tai chi styles. When you are ready to move on, there are videos available from Dr. Lam that can expand your practice (*see Resources, page 139*).

Choosing a tai chi class

No matter how good a book or video, it cannot convey the experience of studying tai chi with a teacher. A teacher can help you by pointing out errors you might be making, and by giving you good advice on how to make your tai chi practice stronger and deeper. Also, many people enjoy attending classes for the social interaction and the pleasure of moving through the tai chi forms in unison with others.

Take care to select a teacher who truly understands the underlying philosophy of tai chi and who has experience of teaching people with a wide range of abilities. Some who say they are teaching tai chi may not have had proper training, either in tai chi or in sports medicine. Many teachers over-emphasize the martial arts aspects, which can be harmful to people with musculoskeletal problems.

Qualities to look for in a teacher

Tai chi is an art of immense depth. It has become very popular, so there may be a shortage of qualified teachers in some places. Also, there is no standard certification for tai chi teachers. You may contact Dr. Lam (*see Resources, page 139*) for a list of instructors who have experience in tai chi for arthritis in your area.

A knowledge of tai chi

Classes may be taught by someone who is not expert in tai chi. Before signing up for a class, do some research by checking the reputation of teachers in your community.

Experience of working with people with arthritis

Even an exercise programme as gentle as tai chi can be harmful if it is not practised properly. Be sure the teacher has experience of working with people who also have your kind of arthritis.

Ask your doctor or physiotherapist to recommend a class. And be sure to tell the teacher about your condition and any movements that are difficult, uncomfortable or painful for you.

A teaching method that is comfortable for you

In former times, tai chi teaching was usually one-way communication: the teachers demonstrated the movements, told the students what to do and made the students copy them.

You may be more comfortable with a coaching style of teaching in which you can ask questions about matters which have particular relevance to you. Good teachers make sure they know the limits of every student in their class and are careful not to go beyond these. You should feel able to stop and ask your instructor to explain the movements and to suggest adaptations that will take into account your symptoms.

Patience and understanding

Find a teacher who is not in a hurry and who will patiently listen to your concerns. Tai chi takes time for anyone to learn and people with a mobility problem or who are in pain may take much longer.

DANGER SIGNS

You may have tried tai chi and found it painful, or that it had no effect on your arthritis symptoms. Unfortunately, you may not have been getting proper instruction. Perhaps you were trying a form of tai chi too stressful for your physical condition. Here are some warning signs to find another class:

IF THE TEACHER SAYS "NO PAIN, NO GAIN"

Research has shown this old myth is not only untrue, but dangerous. You can benefit from exercise without aching. In fact, exercise should not hurt, except for some mild discomfort at first or when moving to a more demanding level. And that discomfort should not last more than a few hours afterwards.

IF THE TEACHER ASKS YOU TO ASSUME AN EXTREME STRETCH

In exercise terms, more can sometimes be dangerous. Extreme stretches can leave you sore and may even cause damage. Stretch slowly only to within a comfortable range.

IF THE TEACHER ASKS YOU TO "BOUNCE" INTO A STRETCH

Muscles that are stressed with short, jerky motions don't stretch out and relax – they actually get tighter with every bounce, so you end up straining them. Stretches should be eased into gradually and held without moving for 2 to 10 seconds.

Useful arthritis organizations

Arthritis Research Campaign
St Mary's Court, St Mary's Gate, Chesterfield,
Derbs S41 7TD
Phone: 01246 558033
Fax: 01246 558007
E-mail: info@arc.org.uk
Website: www.arc.org.uk
Publishes the magazine *Arthritis Today*.

Arthritis Care (UK)
18 Stephenson Way, London NW1 2HD
Phone: 020 7380 6500
Freephone Helpline: 0808 800 4050
Fax: 020 7380 6505
Web. www.arthritiscare.org.uk
Publishes the magazine *Arthritis News*.

The British Society for Rheumatology
41 Eagle St., London WC1R 4AR
Phone: 020 7242 3313
Fax: 020 7242 3277
Email: bsr@rheumatology.org.uk

**Lady Hoare Trust for Physically Disabled
Children**
1st Floor, 89 Albert Embankment,
London SE1 7TP
Phone: 020 7820 9989
Fax: 020 7582 8251
E-mail: info@lhtchildren.org.uk
Website: www.ladyhoaretrust.org.uk

The Arthritis Foundation of Ireland
1 ClanWilliam Square, Grand Canal Quay,
Dublin 2, Ireland.
Phone: +353 1 661 8188
Fax: +353 1 661 6261

E-mail: info@arthritis-foundation.com
Website: www.arthritis-foundation.com

**University of Birmingham Department
of Rheumatology**
Website: www.rheumb.bham.ac.uk

The Horder Centre for Arthritis
St John's Rd., Crowborough, Sussex TN6 1XP
Phone: 01892 665577
Fax: 01892 662142
E-mail: arthritis@horder.co.uk
Website: www.arthritisathorder.com

National Osteoporosis Society (NOS)
Camerton, Bath BA2 0PJ
Phone: 01761 471771 (for general enquiries)
Helpline: 01761 472721 (for medical queries)
Fax: 01761 471104
E-mail: info@nos.org.uk
Website: www.nos.org.uk

Lupus UK
1 Eastern Rd., Romford, Essex RM1 3NH
Tel: 01708 731251 Fax: 01708 731252

The Psoriatic Arthropathy Alliance (PAA)
Contact: David Chandler
PO Box 111, St Albans, Herts, AL2 3JQ
Phone/fax: 0870 703212
E-mail: office@paalliance.org
Website: www.paalliance.org

Psoriatic Arthritis Liaison Scotland
Contact: J. Johnson
54 Bellevue Rd., Edinburgh, EH7 4DE
Phone: 0131 556 4117

Tai Chi for Arthritis teachers & videos

Rising Moon Tai Chi Ch'uan
Contact: Derek Williamson
48 Moss Rd., Tillicoultry, Scotland FK13 6NS
Phone: 07973 684182
E-mail: enquiries@risingmoontaichi.com
Website: www.risingmoontaichi.com

The Tai Chi & Chi Kung Forum for Health and Special Needs
Contact: Linda Chase Broda
c/o 163 Palatine Road, Manchester M20 2GH
Phone: 0161 445 1568
E-mail: forum@connectfree.co.uk
Website: www.taichiandspecialneeds.co.uk

The Tai Chi Union for Great Britain
1 Littlemill Drive, Balmoral Gardens
Crookston, Glasgow G53 7GE, Scotland
Phone: 0141 810 3482
Fax: 0141 810 3741
E-mail: secretary@taichiunion.com
Website: www.taichiunion.com

White Crane Taijiquan
Contact: Mandeigh Wells
10 Glebe Rd., Kinloss, Scotland IV36 3TU
Phone: 01309 690272
E-mail: mandeigh@bigfoot.com
Website: www.taijiscotland.org.uk

Tai Chi Cambridge
Contact: Mike Tabrett
6 Swanns Terrace, Cambridge CB1 3LX
Phone: 01223 503390
Fax: 0709 331927
E-mail: Mike@taichicambridge.co.uk
Website: www.taichicambridge.co.uk

Other useful UK resource sites:
www.taichifinder.co.uk (UK directory, includes style comments).

www.taichiforarthritis.com (information on the programme and a list of certified teachers).

Videos
Dr. Lam's best-selling video, Tai Chi for Arthritis, takes you through the sequences step-by-step and is available in English, Chinese, French and Spanish as a DVD and in English and Chinese as a video.

Dr. Paul Lam's team of experts have produced several other tai chi videos that range from introductory "teach yourself" series for health, arthritis and better lifestyle, to the advanced series which expand your skill. All videos are available in NTSC or PAL format, and are sold on Dr. Lam's website (see address below). The following are the more popular titles:
Tai Chi for Arthritis Part II
Tai Chi for Diabetes
Tai Chi for Older Adults (over 55)
Qigong for Health
Tai Chi Anywhere
Tai Chi for Young People

For mail, phone, online and e-mail orders:
4 Fisher Place, Narwee NSW 2209 Australia
Phone: 61 2 9533 6511; or 61 2 9534 4311
Fax: 61 2 9534 4311
E-mail: service@taichiproductions.com
Website: www.taichiproductions.com

Further reading

Following is our list of recommended books in order of priority:

The Arthritis Foundation's Guide to Alternative Therapies Judith Horstman (Arthritis Foundation, Atlanta, 1999)

Taijiquan Chen style 36 Forms Professor Kan Gui Xiang and Dr. Paul Lam (East Acton Publishing, Sydney, 1992)

Xing Yi Quan Xue, The Study of Form – Mind Boxing Sun Lu Tang, trans. by Albert Liu, compiled and edited by Dan Miller (High View Publication, 1993)

The Essence of T'ai Chi Ch'uan – The Literary Tradition trans. and edited by Benjamin Pang Jeng Lo; Martin Inn; Robert Amacker; and Susan Foe (North Atlantic Books, Berkeley, California, 1979)

The Arthritis Helpbook: A Tested Self-Management Program for Coping with Arthritis and Fibromyalgia (Fifth Edition) Kate Lorig, RN, DrPH, and James F. Fries, MD (Perseus Books, Reading, Massachusetts, 2000)

The Inner Structure of Tai Chi Chia, Mantak and Juan Li (Healing Tao Books, Huntington, NY, 1996)

Ride the Tiger to the Mountain – Tai Chi for Health Martin Lee, Emily Lee and JoAn Johnstone (Perseus Books, Reading, Massachusetts, 1989)

Health Quotient Dr Tze (Random House, Canada, 2001)

Exercise Beats Arthritis Valerie Sayce and Ian Fraser (Fraser Publications, Victoria, Australia, 1987)

Arthritis – Your Complete Exercise Guide Neil Gordon (Human Kinetics, Champaign, Illinois, 1993)

Simplified Taijiquan China Sports Series 1, compiled by China Sports Editorial Board, Beijing, China, 1980

Yang Style Taijiquan Morning Glory Press (Hai Feng Publishing Co, Hong Kong, 1988)

The Complete Idiot's Guide to Tai Chi and QiGong Bill Douglas and Richard Yennie (Alpha Books, New York, 1999)

Chen Style Taijiquan compiled by Zhaohua Publishing House, Hong Kong (Hai Feng Publishing Co, 1984)

Taiji: 48 Forms and Swordplay China Sports Series 3, compiled by China Sports Editorial Board, Beijing, China, 1988

Cheng Man-Ch'ing's Advanced T'ai-Chi Form Instructions compiled and translated by Douglas Wile (Sweet Chi Press, Brooklyn, NY, 1985)

Tai Chi Ch'uan – The Technique of Power Tem Horwitz and Susan Kimmelman (Rider and Company, London, 1979)

Embrace Tiger, Return To Mountain Chung Liang Al Huang (Celestial Arts, Berkeley, California, 1997)

Chinese Qigong Massage, General Massage Jwing–Ming Yang (YMAA Publication Center, Jamaica Plain, Massachusetts, 1992)

Full Catastrophe Living: Using the wisdom of your body and mind to face stress, pain and illness Jon Kabat–Zinn (Delta Books, New York, 1990)

8 Weeks to Optimum Health: A Proven Program for Taking Full Advantage of Your Body's Natural Healing Power Andrew Weil, MD (Fawcett Books, New York, 1998)

Foods That Fight Pain Neal Barnard, MD (Harmony Books, New York, 1998)

Index

A page number in **bold** indicates a main entry on a topic.

AUTHORS' ACKNOWLEDGEMENTS

We are grateful to the thousands of
people with arthritis and to the tai chi
instructors who inspired and helped
develop this programme, and to arthritis
organizations worldwide, including the
Arthritis Foundation of Australia and
the Arthritis Foundation of the USA.

We would also like to thank:

Tony Coyle for supporting this book;
Valerie Sayce and Dr. Terry Kwong for
editing and review; and Anna Bennett,
practice manager for the Tai Chi for
Arthritis programme.

Our families, for their love and support. And especially Mr. Win Gwai Lum,
Dr. Lam's father-in-law and first teacher,
who is still practising tai chi and enjoying
great health at age 89.

**PUBLISHER'S
ACKNOWLEDGEMENTS**

Dorling Kindersley would like to thank
the following people for their help and
participation in this project:
Claudia Mitchell, Rosemary McDonald,
Carla Masson and Sue Bosanko.

THE TAI CHI FOR ARTHRITIS TEAM

The Tai Chi for Arthritis programme was developed by:

* Paul Lam, family doctor and tai chi expert.
* Tai chi instructors Julie King, Michael Ngai, Robyn Nicholls and Ian Etcell.
* Professor John Edmonds MBBS, MFRACP, Conjoint Professor of Rheumatology at the University of New South Wales and Head of Rheumatology Department, St. George Hospital, Sydney.
* Dr. Ian Portek MBBS, MFRACP, spokesman for Arthritis Foundation of New South Wales, and a rheumatologist in Sydney.
* Guni Hinchey, Senior Rheumatology Physiotherapist, St. George Hospital, Sydney.

PICTURE CREDITS

Picture Researcher: Samantha Nunn
Picture Librarians: Richard Dabb and David Saldanha

The publisher would like to thank the following for their kind permission to reproduce their photographs:
(Abbreviations key: t=top, b=bottom, r=right, l=left, c=centre)

Pictor International: 13.
Science Photo Library: Paul Biddle 63b; Paul Biddle & Tim Malyon 67tr; CNRI 20t; Mehau Kulyk 59b; Dr P. Marazzi 22bl; Prof P. Motta/Dept. of Anatomy/University of "La Sapienza", Rome 55br; Dr Yorgos Nikas 60l; Princess Margaret Rose Orthopaedic Hospital 61r; Sean O'Brien, Custom Medical Stock Photo 40t.
Corbis Stock Market: 51b; Rick Gomez 2; Larry Williams 15b.
Stone/Getty Images: 45t, 84t, 91tr.
Telegraph Colour Library/Getty Images: 27, 42b, 89b.
Alcina Horstman: 9.

Jacket Picture Credits
ImageState: back jacket tl.
Stone/Getty Images: back jacket clb.

ILLUSTRATION CREDITS

Richard Tibbitts: 17, 19.
Jörn Kroger 10, 24, 48, 74, 86, 102.
All other images © Dorling Kindersley.

For further information see:
www.dkimages.com

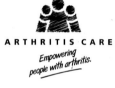

ARTHRITIS CARE
Empowering people with arthritis.

Arthritis Care is the largest UK-wide voluntary organization working with and for all people with arthritis. It aims to empower people to take control of their arthritis and their lives. The organization has 45,000 members and nearly 600 branches and groups throughout the UK.

Arthritis Care offers a wide range of services to people with arthritis. It provides a confidential helpline service by letter and telephone Monday to Friday, 12 noon to 4pm, on a freephone helpline (080 8800 4050). The service is also available from Monday to Friday, 10am to 4pm, when calls are charged at the national rate (020 7380 6555).

The Source is Arthritis Care's helpline service for young people with arthritis. Contact it by letter, telephone (freephone 080 8808 2000 Monday to Friday, 10am to 2pm and Monday, 4pm to 7pm) or by email: *thesource@arthritiscare.org.uk*

Arthritis Care is considered a leader in the field of self-management. It offers a range of self-management and personal development training courses for people with arthritis of all ages to enable them to be in control of their arthritis.

Arthritis Care improves access to information about arthritis through a range of helpful and informative publications, covering issues such as independent living, diet, exercise, medication and complementary therapies. It also publishes a bi-monthly magazine, *Arthritis News,* which covers all aspects of living with arthritis.

Arthritis Care campaigns actively for greater awareness of the needs of all people with arthritis, including their needs for treatment and access. The organization also runs four hotels in the UK, all equipped to make sure the needs and comfort of people with arthritis are catered for.

For a free information pack about Arthritis Care and the services it offers, ring the 24-hour information line on 0845 6006868. Or visit the website at: *www.arthritiscare.org.uk*